Surviving Mental Illness

SURVIVING MENTAL ILLNESS

Stress, Coping, and Adaptation

AGNES B. HATFIELD
HARRIET P. LEFLEY

Foreword by John S. Strauss

THE GUILFORD PRESS
New York   London

ABA 1734

©1993 The Guilford Press
A Division of Guilford Publications, Inc.
72 Spring Street, New York, NY 10012

Printed in the United States of America

This book is printed on acid-free paper.

Last digit is print number: 9 8 7 6 5 4 3 2 1

Library of Congress Cataloging-in-Publication Data
Hatfield, Agnes B.
    Surviving mental illness: stress, coping, and adaptation / Agnes
B. Hatfield, Harriet P. Lefley.
        p.   cm.
    Includes bibliographical references and index.
    ISBN 0-89862-124-0.   ISBN 0-89862-022-8 (pbk.)
    1. Mental illness. 2. Mentally ill—Attitudes. 3. Chronically
ill—Attitudes. 4. Adaptation (Psychology) 5. Social psychiatry.
I. Lefley, Harriet P. II. Title.
    [DNLM: 1. Stress, Psychological—psychology. 2. Adaptation,
Psychological. 3. Mental Disorders—psychology. WM 100 H362s
1993]
    616.89—dc20
    DNLM/DLC
    for Library of Congress   93-20492
                                                                 CIP

Foreword

"Is it like a voice—or a thought?" I asked the person with schizophrenia with whom I was conducting the research interview. Trying to differentiate whether this person had delusions or hallucinations or both, I was asking the usual questions. "Well, not really either. It's kind of like a thought, but it's stronger than that, almost like a voice," he replied. He had not yet learned that he was supposed to shape the description of his experiences to fit the concepts that we professionals use. Or perhaps he was merely trying to be true to his experience. Maitland Baldwin had taught me years ago how patients with epilepsy, after repeating their medical histories numerous times, learn to tell their stories to fit the questions that professionals ask. The same tends to happen in a variety of mental disorders.

It is only from the most neutral inquiry, and, even more likely, from the kinds of autobiographical material that Drs. Hatfield and Lefley have collected here, that we really can come closer to understanding the nature of mental disorders. And the word "understanding" has powerful implications. It includes empathy, feeling with, understanding what someone who has a particular experience is going through and how it might affect the way he or she views the world and attempts to deal with it. "Understanding" also includes treatment, to improve the ability to help a person with a particular kind of experience and monitor improvement or worsening in a way that fits with his or her reality. "Understanding" includes research, so that research focuses not on the causes, for example, of just voices or of just delusions, when in fact the real phenomena are more complex. A rating scale that asks only the questions of a particular profession, even of a particular era in the field, perhaps poorly fitted to the real experiences of a real person, or a biological test to fit only the roughest approximation of a phenomenon that the person experiences, is far less likely to be useful and productive than a rating scale or a biological test that links closely to the experience as it exists.

And understanding the nature of mental disorders in a way that reflects the experience of the person also has implications for theory. Labels and explanations for phenomena depend closely for their accuracy and helpfulness on careful attention to what those phenomena are. Currently, the belief that "it's all basically biological" has superseded the belief of only a couple of decades ago that "it's all basically because of the society," which superseded the belief of the decades before that "it's all because of the family." Each of these beliefs has been based on readings of the data considered relevant at the time, but it seems to me that any one of these conclusions alone goes far beyond the evidence provided by the findings available. And yet, to the extent that we do extend our beliefs beyond the data, our theories become more and more questionable, and our certainties may prevent us from seeing the entirety or the complexity of the truth. I personally believe, for example, that the psychological and experiential can have as much impact on the biological as the reverse, and the arrows of cause in severe mental disorder involve a wide range of complex sequences of direction and interaction, most of which we do not yet understand. The starting points are far from clear. But no matter what theory or theories are eventually found to be correct, such discovery will depend on the dictum that, like the customer, "the patient is always right." A concept like hallucinations or a theory of schizophrenia and its causes will depend ultimately on learning what people with mental disorders really experience. Whenever we forget to listen carefully or lose cognizance of observer bias—the ways we shape what we see and record— forgetting, for example, to note the feelings and the competence as well as the problems of people with disorders, we push ourselves that much farther from finding the answer.

The accounts provided by Drs. Hatfield and Lefley in this volume move in a crucial direction, toward a clearer understanding in all regards of the nature of severe mental disorders. And as we—"patients," "nonpatients," "consumers," "nonconsumers"—struggle with these problems, it is up to each of us to separate what comprises data—the direct reports of experience and the observations of experiences and behaviors— from the many theories, past, present, and future, that reflect our efforts at understanding. Theories can provide understanding or distortion; the ultimate truth is in the data.   .

JOHN S. STRAUSS, M.D.
Department of Psychiatry
Yale University

Introduction

The focus of this book is on the experiential side of the major mental illnesses. Although the psychiatric field has progressed substantially in the past few decades in understanding the biology of mental illness and in developing appropriate psychopharmacological treatments, few would claim that we have advanced as far in our understanding of the inner world of people experiencing these illnesses. The few books that have been written about this inner world in the past have used a psychodynamic framework to assign a meaning and purpose to symptomatology. There has been little effort to understand how persons experience psychiatric disability in a society that demeans their condition, or in a helping environment that only dimly understands their agony. Yet increasing our capacity for empathy, developing more effective rehabilitation strategies, and advancing research that links brain anomalies and patients' experience depend, in large part, upon our ability to understand the patients' subjective experience. Leading researchers such as John Strauss of Yale University and William Carpenter of the Maryland Psychiatric Research Institute have noted in their work the importance of understanding this neglected area of investigation.

Significant interest in the inner world of mental illness is beginning to emerge in all the core mental health disciplines. Leading psychiatric journals such as *Schizophrenia Bulletin* and *Hospital and Community Psychiatry* now feature first-person accounts of patients' experiences. Consumers of mental health services are often invited to be presenters at major professional meetings, and their sessions are invariably well attended. Our impressions, from participation in a variety of national conferences, is that professionals have a keen interest in knowing more about the phenomenal side of mental illness.

Fortunately, there is a large accumulation of first-person accounts in a wide diversity of resources—consumer newsletters, informal communications, professional journals, and books written by former patients. There are also findings from a very few scientific surveys that actually delve into how mental illness is experienced by adequately large and representative samples of this group of citizens. This book is an effort to weave together, from the spoken presentations, writings, research reports, and observed behaviors of people who have suffered from psychiatric disabilities, some common patterns in the lifetime experience of severe and persistent mental illness.

In contrast to earlier works that have used a traditional psychodynamic rationale for "understanding" mental illness, this book subscribes to the contemporary view of major psychiatric disorders as biologically based disease entities that have strong social and psychological meaning to the subject. Our conceptual framework, based largely on coping and adaptation theory, is discussed in greater detail in Chapter 2. Using this framework, we have tried to derive from the written, spoken, and behavioral products of consumers a picture of how mentally ill people cope with, and how some are able to transcend, their various disabilities.

The themes discussed in the book as a whole are the responsibility of the authors. As behavioral scientists and university professors, we have used the skills of our disciplines to derive patterns and themes from the writings of multiple consumers. We also bring our observations as family members, as long-time participants in the consumer advocate movement, as educators, and as clinicians or clinical observers. In addition, we have called on the insights of three articulate and knowledgable consumers, two of whom are trained mental health professionals who work with seriously mentally ill people, to describe their particular experiences. Although no consumers speak for all, we believe that the three sensitively written statements in this book are highly educational regarding the meaning of psychosis and hospitalization, the way in which a person with mental illness perceives the interpersonal environment, and the factors conducive to recovery.

For the readers of this book, several cautions must be emphasized. First, many of the materials tend to focus on schizophrenia, since both the research literature and personal recollections of psychotic states have dealt with schizophrenia to a greater extent than with other severe psychiatric conditions. However, the experiences described in these pages reflect those of persons with mulitple diagnoses: schizophrenia, bipolar illness, major endogenous depression, and other disorders with psychotic features and long-term disabling consequences. There is heterogeneity both between and within diagnostic categories—great differences in degree of thought disorder, cognitive and perceptual deficits, and level of disability. People differ not only in their functional capabilities, but in their emotional and rational assessment of their experiences.

The second caution is that even among people who share the same level of functioning, there may be great differences regarding the salience, importance, and evaluation of what happened to them and why. In the multiple first-person accounts, some consumers focus exclusively on the phenomenology of the psychotic episode, while others write mostly about their experiences with the community, their families, or the mental health system. Although most individuals writing about psychosis focus on the terrifying aspects, some also recall special enlightenment and growth. For many consumers, recollections of their experiences in the service delivery system are negative, particularly under conditions of involuntary commitment. But some individuals feel they were a threat to themselves or others, and state publicly that they are thankful they were forced into accepting treatment.

Finally, we have also used coping and adaptation theory, together with some psychodynamic insights, as an explanatory model for behaviors commonly seen and reported by family members and service providers as well as by patients themselves. Many of these behaviors are negative or aversive. They are characteristic sometimes of the symptomtology of major mental illnesses, but more often of patients' reactions to their illnesses and to themselves. They reflect a defensive stance vis-à-vis a critical society, as well as reactions toward professionals and sometimes families and friends who are perceived as uncaring or obstructive.

Service providers often see patients when they are acting negatively rather than positively. It is important for direct care staff members and other caregivers to recognize that coping and adaptation have many facets, and that an adaptive response to mental illness is sometimes initiated by behaviors reflecting rebellion and a search for control. It is even more important to recognize the strengths in patients that can be reinforced by sensitive caregivers to facilitate improvement or recovery. To this end, we have focused in the latter part of this book on lessons from consumers on how professionals, service providers, caregivers, and the community at large can be most helpful to patients in the process of coping and living with major mental illness.

AGNES B. HATFIELD
HARRIET P. LEFLEY

Contents

I. OVERVIEW

1. The Personal Side of Mental Illness   **3**

The Personal Side in Psychosocial Treatments, 4
Families and the Personal Side of Mental Illness, 7
The Role of the Subjective Experience in Research, 8
Summary, 10

**2. A Conceptual Basis for Understanding Patients'
Behavior: The Case of Schizophrenia**   **11**

Stressors and Stress, 13
Coping and Adaptation, 15
Coping Strategies in Schizophrenia, 20
Summary and Conclusions, 25

II. HOW PATIENTS EXPERIENCE PSYCHOSIS

3. Disturbances in the Sense of Self   **29**

Disturbed Perception as a Primary Factor, 29
The Loss of a Sense of Self, 30
Altered Sense of Self, 33
Disorders of Attention, 35
Person–Disorder Interactions, 37
Summary, 40

4. Disturbances in Cognition   **42**

Racing Thoughts and Stimulus Overload, 43
Yielding to Associative Connections, 45
Slowed Thoughts and Mental Blocking, 46
Disturbances in Judgment and Reasoning, 48
How Patients Cope with Impaired Cognitive Processes, 49
Implications for Research and Practice, 51
Summary, 54

5. Disturbances in Emotions, Relationships,
   and Behaviors   55
   Disturbances in Emotions, 55
   Disturbances in Relationships and Behaviors, 62
   Implications for Research and Practice, 66

6. Cruising the Cosmos, Part Three: Psychosis and
   Hospitalization—A Consumer's Personal Recollection   67
   Frederick J. Frese, III, Ph.D.

III. HOW PATIENTS EXPERIENCE
THE INTERPERSONAL ENVIRONMENT

7. Patients' Perceptions of Families   79
   How Professionals Have Viewed Families, 80
   Mental Illness in the Family: General Problems
      and Reactions, 81
   Reactions of Siblings and Adult Children, 82
   Patients and Parents: The Critical Issue of Dependency, 84
   Patients' Negative or Conflicted Perceptions of Families, 85
   Patients' Positive Perceptions of Families, 86
   Summary and Conclusions, 89

8. Patients' Perceptions of Professionals and
   the Service Provider System   91
   Patient–Staff Relationships in the Hospital, 91
   Relationships with Professionals in the Community, 93
   Patients' Positive Feelings toward Service Providers
      and Hospitals, 96

9. Community Acceptance and Self-Perception   100
   Housing and Employment, 102
   Societal Restrictions: The Catch-22 Phenomenon, 104
   Internalizing Stigma, 104
   Coping with Stigma: Maladaptive and Adaptive Strategies, 105
   Fighting the Power of Pejorative Language, 107
   Building Community Support, 109
   Summary, 112

10. The Interpersonal Environment—A Consumer's
    Personal Recollection   114
    Esso Leete

    My Early History and the Beginnings of My Illness, 114
    The Importance of the Interpersonal Environment, 118
    Working toward Recovery: Needs and Goals, 125

IV. HOW PATIENTS EXPERIENCE
THE RECOVERY PROCESS

11. Events Leading to Recovery   **131**

Stress, Coping, and Adaptation, 132
Patients' Perceptions of Factors in Recovery, 134
Summary and Implications, 141

**12. Developing an Acceptable Identity and
New Purposes in Life**   **143**

Obstacles to Achieving an Acceptable Identity, 144
Finding Meaning in Life, 147
Summary and Implications, 152

13. Learning to Manage the Illness and Avoid Relapse   **154**

Psychodynamic Issues in Illness Management, 154
Self-Education and Educating Others, 156
Self-Monitoring and Symptom Management, 157
Interaction of Biological Needs and Illness
   Management Strategies, 162
Patients' Organizations in Illness Management, 163
How the System Can Help Patients Help Themselves, 166
Summary and Conclusions, 168

**14. Life on the Ledge: My Recovery from a Major Mental
Illness—A Consumer's Personal Recollection**   **169**
Daniel Link, M.S.W.

V. LESSONS LEARNED FROM CONSUMERS

15. Summary, Conclusions, and Implications   **177**

The Experience of Psychosis, 178
Perceptions of Caregiving and Treatment, 181
Perceptions of the Recovery Process, 184
Thoughts on Future Directions, 187

References   **189**

Index   **201**

Surviving Mental Illness

SECTION ONE

OVERVIEW

CHAPTER ONE

The Personal Side
of Mental Illness

During a period of significant advances in many aspects of psychiatry, we have made little progress in our understanding of what it is like to be the person who is suffering from a debilitating mental illness. In the past, psychiatrists have used a host of historical, mythical, and literary characters to illuminate the nature of these disorders, but rarely the experiences of those so afflicted. We ignore the fact that they are insiders in the experience of mental illness and we are outsiders (Sommer & Osmond, 1961). Carpenter (1986), who has given significant attention to the experiential side of mental illness in his writings, has said:

> The most irreducible essence of our interest in schizophrenia is the nature of another person's experience. It is in the subjective and inner world of volition, perception, cognition, and affect that schizophrenia is manifest. Empathy is crucial in discovering the subjective life of another person, and to engage in this process with a psychotic person, requires skill, intuition, and perseverance. (p. 534)

In a journal article entitled "Are Psychiatric Educators 'Losing the Mind'?," Reiser (1988) deplored psychiatric educators' lack of curiosity about the patient as a person. He felt that most of the residents he knew could or would have learned more about a stranger sitting next to them on an airplane than they chose to learn about their patients as human beings. For Reiser this indicated a serious flaw in training.

Those who suffer from these illnesses also express displeasure at being only objects of treatment and never being fully understood. McGrath (1984), reacting to the excesses of technological explanations, has stated:

3

> I suddenly feel that my humanity has been sacrificed to a computer printout, that the researchers have dissected me without realizing that I am still alive. I am not comfortable or safe in all their certain uncertainties. . . . I feel they are losing me, the person, more and more. (p. 639)

Making a similar point upon the recovery from a serious mental illness, Brundage (1983) has concluded: "The effectiveness in reaching and working with patients rests largely upon the ability of the caregiver to perceive and comprehend how particular patients are experiencing their illnesses" (p. 585). Only in this way can we give feedback that is understandable to patients in their world, and in other ways be helpful to them.

In a newsletter called *Hang Tough*, published by the Marin Network of Mental Health Clients, Stephen Weiner (1985) has talked about the mental health consumer movement and its likely consequences:

> We make a radical demand, one of the most difficult to fulfill: we insist that people get inside our heads and skins and try to empathize. This is something that all outsider groups have demanded, yet the experience of psychosis may be the most forbidding of all. Our plea cannot be "we're just like you" because that isn't true. On the other hand it's not completely untrue. (p. 3)

Better understanding of the personal side of mental illness can lead to more effective work with patients in clinics and rehabilitation centers, as well as with their families. In can also lead to better research, for as Schwartz and Wiggins (1985) point out, all science arises out of the prescientific experiences of everyday life. The prescientific experience of reality is never erased by science, though science reaches beyond it.

THE PERSONAL SIDE
IN PSYCHOSOCIAL TREATMENTS

Mendel (1974) and Carpenter (1986) view phenomenology as the crucial concept in clinical psychiatry and decry the shallowness of purely descriptive approaches in treatment. Mendel has noted the limitations in such often-used clinical descriptions as "thought-process disorder," "impaired reality testing," "shallow interpersonal relationships," and "defective ego functioning." Although these terms may be useful in certain kinds of professional communication, they convey nothing of a patient's inner experience. At best, they describe the person's symptoms, but they do not increase empathetic understanding. What is more, such descriptions may serve as a substitute for genuine empathic understanding and preclude clinicians' continued efforts to get into the experiences of their patients.

Clinical observation is the backbone of scientific medicine. In psychiatric disorders, where the core disturbance is manifested in altered subjective experiences, it is important to know how patients conceptualize their experiences and their expectations for care. Clinicians must be able to make contact and get information relevant to overall functioning, including adequacy of ego functioning and the capacity for establishing relationships (Carpenter & Hanlon, 1986).

Clinicians must learn to deal with the disruption of identity, for questions of identity have great urgency to the patient: "Who am I? Can I relate? What will become of me? Have I damaged others?" Patients often believe that their experiences are too incomprehensible to share, and they maintain secret fears about them. Clinicians may prefer to ignore the "craziness," but patients may be immensely reassured by knowing that others know their inner world (Carpenter & Hanlon, 1986).

A patient's insight into his or her illness is typically considered important for engagement in treatment and for an adequate prognosis. However, research into insight has not been pursued to determine whether it plays a part in treatment outcome. In fact, there is no agreed-upon definition of "insight." The concept appears to be employed to indicate the degree to which patients believe that they have a mental illness. Lack of insight is equated with denial. We need to understand much more about the range of viewpoints that patients have about their particular dilemmas and how they explain their illness to themselves. Greenfield, Strauss, Bowers, and Mandelkern (1989) did interview studies and found that patients held a wide range of viewpoints about their illness. Their explanations tended toward complexity; this raised questions about earlier studies (e.g., McGlashan & Carpenter, 1976; McGlashan, Levy, & Carpenter, 1975), which used two major poles ("integration" and "sealing over") to define patient insight.

Lally (1989) has stressed the importance of knowing the patients' struggles to define themselves. He has drawn upon labeling theory (Goffman, 1961) to explore the role of labels in the destruction of self-concept, with particular emphasis on the way patients label themselves. Hospitals contribute to the loss of the person by defining people as psychiatric patients. Lally has used the term "engulfment" to describe the condition in which a patient's concept is significantly organized around the patient role. He speculates that a total acceptance of the disorder may compound patient passivity. Lally recommends that the costs and benefits of different responses to the illness be studied.

Lehman (1982, 1988) has done considerable research on quality-of-life issue for patients, and has concluded that listening to what patients have to say about their lives can provide useful insights into types of services needed. The literature provides considerable evidence that patients often have perspectives on treatment differing from those of service providers. According to Lehman, if a provider overlooks or underestimates problems perceived by a patient as important, noncompliance is probable.

In addition to noteworthy concerns for client preferences and needs for services, psychiatric rehabilitation services might profitably give more attention to the inner world of their clients—how they see their particular dilemmas in life and the nature of their personal struggles for a meaningful existence. Strauss (1986) sees a great deal of potential for the field of psychiatric rehabilitation, and feels that we may be underestimating what it contributes to the actual healing process. What are not clear, Strauss notes, are the nature and origins of these processes of improvement.

Strauss (1986) believes that important processes found in clinical studies of mentally ill persons may be of help in rehabilitation. These processes are the efforts that a person makes in his or her own recovery, the role of meanings, and the sense of identity. The person himself or herself is an important factor in the course and outcome of the illness. Summarizing the work of a number of researchers, Strauss concludes that people play an important role in controlling their own symptoms and in selecting and using the kinds of help available. They choose to collaborate with treatment, to seek out or avoid social supports, and to withdraw or take risks in their own behalf. Rehabilitation, with its potential for helping people to become goal-directed and to develop a socially accepted identity, can work with the strengths of these individuals and can play a significant role in eventual outcome.

Given the strength of the argument for more empathic understanding of patients, it is important to ask why such understanding is not as widespread as it should be. Minkoff and Stern (1985) believe that for most clinicians schizophrenia is a terrifying disease, and that "the devastation, shame, and despair of the experience of chronic psychosis makes [sic] empathy very painful even for the most experienced clinician, let alone the trainee" (p. 863). Not only is it difficult to make a connection with the person behind the psychosis, but once the connection is made, the patient's despair at having a chronic mental illness may be more than the clinician can tolerate.

Sarason (1985) says that the world view into which mental health trainees are initiated renders them insensitive to the phenomenological plight of the individuals they are expected to help. Sarason feels that there has been too much emphasis on objectivity and too much worry about "emotional involvement." As additional barriers, he identifies our large bureaucratic institutions, the way we select students for admission to mental health training, and the overemphasis on technical skill. Sarason emphasizes that caring and compassion involve pain, inconvenience, and self-sacrifice. Understanding of another comes through grappling with three obstacles: underestimation of the scope and complexity of the problem, failure to use one's life experiences creatively, and resistance to the idea that the process is unending.

FAMILIES AND THE PERSONAL SIDE OF MENTAL ILLNESS

Torrey (1983, 1988) has made an eloquent plea for the importance of families' understanding the "inner world of mental madness," for when tragedy strikes, he explains, one of the things that makes things bearable is the sympathy of friends and relatives. The "prerequisite for sympathy is an ability to put oneself in the place of the person afflicted" (1983, p. 5). Sympathy for those with mental illness is limited, however, because few people are able to fathom what lies behind the bizarre behavior. Torrey has written:

> With sympathy, schizophrenia is a personal tragedy. Without sympathy, it becomes a family calamity, for there is nothing to knit people together, no balm for the wounds. Understanding schizophrenia helps to demystify the disease and brings it from the realm of the occult to the daylight of reason. As we come to understand it, the face of madness slowly changes before us from one of terror to one of sadness. For the sufferer, this is a significant change. (1983, p. 6)

Several books on family education and psychoeducation include an emphasis on teaching families about the personal side of mental illness. Anderson, Reiss, and Hogarty (1986) emphasize in their survival skills workshops the sense of distraction, stimulus overload, sensitivity, and misperception that characterize schizophrenia. Bernheim, Lewine, and Beale (1982) have also given attention to understanding the ill person's experience with mental illness and in guiding families to appropriate responses. More recently, one of us (Hatfield, 1990) has devoted a chapter to the personal side of mental illness in a book on family education. She has used quotations from patients to illustrate altered perceptions, attention deficits, cognitive confusion, and emotional changes. Special emphasis is given to the problems of coming to terms with an altered life, developing an acceptable identity, learning to manage the illness and provide self-care, and coping with stigma.

The National Alliance for the Mentally Ill has published auto-biographical accounts of the patient experience in a short book edited by Shetler and Straw (1982) called *A New Day: Voices from across the Land*. More recently, the National Alliance has published *The Experiences of Patients and Families: First Person Accounts Reprinted from Schizophrenia Bulletin and the New York Times*. A former president of this group, William Snavely (1989) has written in the foreword to the latter publication:

> Accounts of patients and family members of their experiences with mental illness have an authenticity and perspective that cannot be matched by writers who stand outside the ravages of mental illness. Such accounts deepen the understanding of readers who themselves suffer mental illnesses as patients or family members and strengthens their feelings that they are not alone. (p. v)

THE ROLE OF THE SUBJECTIVE EXPERIENCE IN RESEARCH

Most of the information on which we build our understanding about schizophrenia and other major mental disorders comes initially from patient reports. This information gets transformed into technical language by researchers and teachers. The challenge, as Estroff (1989) has noted, is to discover and develop methods that preserve subjectivity.

Patient reports have constituted the data base for descriptive psychiatry from the time of Kraepelin to the creation of the *Diagnostic and Statistical Manual of Mental Disorders* (DSM). We cannot hear or see the delusional experience, so we rely on patients' accounts for validation and for the creation of descriptive categories. We also rely on patients' statements to validate the connection between thought and behavior (Strauss & Estroff, 1989). Many of the logical connections between thought and behavior may be lost because we do not listen to our patients. This failure severely limits the accuracy and validity of current descriptive psychiatry (Strauss, 1989).

Strauss (1989b) feels that research in the experiential side of mental illness has been limited because we are too dominated by specific theories to notice the full range of patient experiences. Another barrier to effective research is the assumption that patient experiences must be translated rapidly into biological or psychological explanations. We must relinquish the feeling that we always know the answers, and we must be willing just to listen for a while with open minds.

Good science requires that we be open to all the data and that we not misleadingly narrow our sources of information. Too often the focus is on static labeling and categorizing. We need to focus on progress and change (Strauss, 1989). Methods of the physical sciences may not be totally applicable for the optimal study of mental life. We need to search for complementary research methods.

Kerlinger (1973), a well-known expert in research methodology, has stated that personal documents are a legitimate source of data. Instead of direct observations of behavior or standardized instruments, written communications are used. With the aid of content analysis, personal documents can be used to test hypotheses. They are thereby considered the same as any other data and are subject to the same rules and laws. In using such documents, we are not doing anything substantially different from observational activities; we are observing and measuring variables.

Kerlinger has also noted, however, that the use of personal documents can present problems of sampling. These accounts cannot be considered unbiased, objective, or representative. As Sommer and Osmond (1960, 1961) have observed, subjectivity is their greatest strength and their greatest weakness. People who write their personal stories tend to be better educated, more literate, and more articulate than other patients. Accounts may also be self-serving to patients: They may provide them with an avenue to see themselves in a good light or to criticize those who have wronged them. But, note Sommer and Osmond, no approach to something as complex, elusive, and difficult to define as mental disorder can be completely objective or unbiased. Combined with other methods, the use of personal documents can be valuable.

Wadeson and Carpenter (1976) reported another approach to learning a patient's perspective on his or her own illness. Patients were asked to draw a number of pictures: a picture of whatever the patients chose, a self-portrait, a picture of their psychiatric illness, and a picture of the hallucinations and delusions experienced. Then they were asked to talk about the illness. Drawings were requested during an acute, drug-free period and 1 year later.

Estroff (1981) studied the everyday life of clients on a 2-year ethnographic field study. By living with them in their world, she learned how they viewed their experiences in the community. This included their views about taking medications, the positive and adverse effects of Supplementary Security Income, and the way they assessed their rehabilitation programs.

Estroff's (1989) current research interests lie in issues related to self and identity. She is interested in how patients represent themselves and in how a person interacts with a disorder. She wonders whether schizophrenia is an "I am" illness that may overtake and redefine the personality. Chronicity may be seen as a loss of self. Estroff is doing continuing research collecting illness–identity statements. Some patients make "I am" statements about their illness, and some make "I have" statements. Estroff is interested in learning whether this has any connection to prognosis.

DeVries and Delespaul (1989) make a strong case for studying responses of patients in a variety of contexts. They feel we need to understand why a person is so remarkably different in different situations. People with schizophrenia are especially vulnerable to fluctuations in their environment: They react more sharply and are less able to maintain homeostatic control; they are less able to stabilize their behavior after a stimulus change; and thought and affect are often influenced. Although this has been frequently observed, we do not know the subjective side of this phenomenon.

SUMMARY

For a variety of reasons, the subjective side of mental illness has been neglected by researchers and educators. There is now a renewed interest in learning about the personal experiences of those who suffer from severe mental disorders. Psychiatric research depends upon the first-person experiences for validation of its findings. Our ability to develop more effective treatment in clinics and more efficacious work in psychiatric rehabilitation depends, in large part, upon more empathic understanding of the people to be served.

CHAPTER TWO

A Conceptual Basis for Understanding Patients' Behavior
The Case of Schizophrenia

For many years, the conceptual framework for understanding the behavior of persons with schizophrenia, bipolar disorder, and other severe psychiatric conditions has been almost exclusively psychodynamic. Major mental illnesses were viewed as arising from a traumatic interpersonal history, and psychotic symptoms presumably represented an idiom of painful metaphors that had to be discovered and reinterpreted to the patient. Behaviors were analyzed as having special psychological meanings, inferred from individual case histories. Major mental illnesses were defined as functional disorders that were psychological in nature and that should be treated primarily by psychological interventions. Rarely if ever was the person afflicted with schizophrenia or manic depression treated as a member of society trying to deal with a disease that had a negative social meaning to the self as well as to others. Rarely was the condition itself perceived as a stressor that required certain coping strategies for the individual to be able to survive.

Although the major diagnostic categories differ in symptoms and presumably in biological substrates, all are perceived by society as mental disorder. In this chapter we use the disease of schizophrenia as an example for understanding patients' behavior in this context. Schizophrenia is viewed here not as a psychogenic disorder, but as a disease process with special personal and social meanings that affect a person's psychological response. Medical sociologists have long pointed out that there is a distinction between "disease," which involves bodily dysfunction, and "illness," which is the patient's experience of the disease. Although most researchers today agree that schizophrenia is indeed a

11

biologically based disease with bodily dysfunction (Nasrallah & Weinberger, 1986), its symptoms are typically observed as deviant behavior
rather than as deviant physiology. Since behavior always has a social
meaning, to the self as well as to others, the disease is therefore experienced as a social phenomenon as well as an illness.

This disease affects its victims in many interrelated contexts, both
internal and external. Internal life is disorganized and fragmented by
the brain dysfunctions, which are manifested behaviorally in aberrant
thinking, misinterpretations of stimuli, and associated terrors. At the
same time, the person with schizophrenia is exposed to ordinary life
events; these may be as typical as missing a bus or being part of a noisy
crowd, but they may be unusually disturbing to persons with the cognitive and perceptual deficits that characterize this particular disorder.

The external context embodies both the patient's perceptions of
himself or herself in relation to others and the interpersonal effects of
schizophrenic behavior. The way the patient processes the reactions of
other people, and the subsequent impact on his or her emotions and
functioning, are important parts of the experience of schizophrenia.
In alerting clinicians to the possibility of their misinterpreting the behavior of their schizophrenic patients, Selzer, Sullivan, Carsky, and Terkelsen (1989) have pointed out:

> The affected individual experiences and manages relationships in
> ways that provoke frequent misunderstanding by a confusion in
> others. To avoid making inaccurate and misleading assumptions, cli-
> nicians must not only understand the disorder but also the individu-
> al's reaction to it. The psychological response to schizophrenia must
> be studied in the patient's manifest and also implied communica-
> tion. (p. 17)

But the person with schizophrenia interacts with many other people in the environment, who are even more likely than clinicians to experience misunderstanding and confusion, and who are considerably
more likely to give negative evaluation feedback than persons who work
with the patient in a therapeutic role. Among the critical questions in
understanding schizophrenic behavior are the extent to which such societal reactions affect the individual's self-concept, and the salience of
the interpersonal situation (behavior of others) as a stressor.

In a revival of the old subjective realism question of whether a tree
actually falls in the forest if it cannot be seen or heard, some authors
have even suggested that mental disorders, unlike physical diseases, cannot exist in isolation from other people. Thus Smoyak (1975), in her
classic psychiatric nursing text, stated: "One can have appendicitis by
himself, but he cannot be paranoid, suicidal, or schizophrenic by him-

self" (p. ix). Smoyak's thinking at the time was that of a family systems framework; it was believed that the mental disorder arose and was maintained in response to a family need for the symptoms. Family causation is disputed today by leading experts in the field, and overviews of research conclude that there is no evidence for this theory of etiology (e.g., Eaton, 1986; Howells & Guirguis, 1985; Liem, 1980; McFarlane & Beels, 1983). Yet there are still a number of commentators who continue to maintain that the behaviors of schizophrenia cannot exist outside of an interpersonal context. This opinion suggests that social responses, rather than the personal terrors, are what sustain the disorder. One of the critical issues in understanding the course of schizophrenic illness—both acute psychosis and chronicity—is the effect of external stress on the internal stimulus events. There are many hypotheses but few empirical models to explain how these variables become processed.

A number of areas of sociological and psychological theory are highly germane to an exploration of schizophrenic behavior. Formerly, we relied almost entirely on psychodynamic and later family systems theories, which have not provided adequate explanatory models for the development of this disorder and have largely ignored the mounting evidence of its biological substrates (Nasrallah & Weinberger, 1986). If we are to achieve a full understanding of schizophrenia as a biopsychosocial phenomenon, the contributions of stress, coping, and adaptation theories; life events research; and self theory must be taken into account. Attribution theory and social role issues are relevant to the intensity and course of illness. Societal tolerance of deviance has been a major theoretical area with respect to the experience of schizophrenia. The deviance hypothesis has ranged from basic etiology—an explanatory model that has lost a great deal of ground but is not yet dead (Barrett, 1989)—to understanding the capacity of persons with schizophrenia to adjust to community living (Sommers, 1987). Cultural world view and attitudes also seem to have an impact on the phenomenological experience and the course of schizophrenic illness (Lefley, 1990). This suggests that under certain conditions, the stressful effects of having a schizophrenic disorder may be mediated by the response of other people in the environment—whether they are members of the treatment staff, family members, friends, or the general public.

STRESSORS AND STRESS

Stress is commonly thought of as a stimulus, an initial triggering event external to the organism. Hans Selye (1976), the father of stress theory, proposed that the external stimulus is actually a "stressor," whereas "stress" is the subsequent physiological disequilibrium of the organism. This condition of stress then becomes an activator of behaviors seeking to resolve the disequilibrium.

Selye seems to have made a spatial distinction between outside stressors and inside stress, but in schizophrenia, both stimulus and response may be internal to the organism. In the framework proposed here, the disease state of brain dysfunction of schizophrenia may be the initial primary stressor that evokes physiological disequilibrium, or internal stress. This disequilibrium then becomes an activator of a series of behavioral responses to internal and external stimulus events.

In generic schizophrenia, as it is currently described in DSM-III-R (American Psychiatric Association, 1987), there may be multiple layers of stressors and stress reactions. We do not know at this point in research the extent to which schizophrenic symptomatology is triggered exclusively by brain dysfunction (a spontaneous aberration of the neurotransmitters), independent of external environmental events. If this possibility is accepted, however, there may be at least two categories of internal stress reactions, primary and secondary — the first spontaneous, the second reactive to external events generated by the first.

Consider the effects of psychotic behavior. Neurotransmitter dysfunction leads to paranoid ideation, which is projected onto another patient, a family member, a case manager, or just someone on the street. The paranoid thought triggers an angry gesture or curse directed toward the object person. The latter feels threatened or offended and reacts with anger. The schizophrenic person feels attacked and decompensates into further paranoid fantasies and perhaps further acting-out behavior. The initial internal stressor, which is physiologically based, has triggered a maladaptive attempt to restore equilibrium by contesting a perceived threat, generating a series of social behaviors with unfortunate consequences.

Smoyak's (1975) statement that schizophrenia cannot be independent of the interpersonal context was predicated on the now-disputed assumption that the behavior of others is a necessary etiological condition for the disease to occur. Our question, however, is whether other people are necessary catalysts for the occurrence of a psychotic reaction. There is considerable evidence in the literature that a variety of life events may trigger decompensation, and among these, interpersonal stressors are frequent but by no means essential conditions (Day et al., 1987). Thus there may be multiple varieties of environmental stimulus events that may trigger a stress reaction, which then becomes an activator of schizophrenic behaviors and their consequences.

Day et al. (1987) found in international research that when

schizophrenic individuals suffered a psychotic episode, they had typically experienced a stressful life event within 3 weeks prior to decompensation. These did not necessarily include other people and were not necessarily negative events. Holmes and Rahe (1967) brought to our attention the notion that life events may be stressors regardless of whether they are objectively pleasant (a wedding, a holiday season) or unpleasant (having an accident, enduring a burglary). For some people, a new baby in the family may be more stressful than losing a job. In all these cases, however, some external event is experienced by the person as something upsetting her or his equilibrium.

Are the symptoms of schizophrenia necessarily stressful to an individual experiencing them? Research by Benjamin (1989) has indicated that auditory hallucinations ("voices") may be perceived as positive (cordial) as well as negative (hostile) by a person with schizophrenia. Are "positive" voices (ranging from nurturing to grandiosity) also perceived as stressors? The complexity of this issue is manifested in Benjamin's suggestion that a cordial relationship between patients and their auditory hallucinations may be adaptive, serving a social-interactional function missing in the social environment. However, "the more adaptive the relationship with the hallucinations, the more intractable and chronic the illness" (p. 308). The assumption here is that interpersonal stress is avoided by substituting an integrated relationship with one's voices for a relationship with other people.

But are "voices" heard in the absence of other people? Certainly a person with schizophrenia is likely to become delusional or to experience hallucinations under conditions that are separate from human transaction: an earthquake or other disaster, homelessness, an accident, or hearing of the death of a loved one. "Voices" are frequently long-term features of the inner environment (North, 1987). They are also likely to appear in the absence of medication, if the individual patient decides that symptoms are preferable to the side effects of the drugs that control the symptoms. Thus we must question whether stress reactions are necessarily responsive to other people, and, in fact, whether they may be totally independent of environmental events. In this connection, we must look at the coping styles and coping strategies that persons with schizophrenia develop in dealing with their disease.

COPING AND ADAPTATION

Hatfield (1987a) has noted that adaptation theory is based on evolutionary concepts, primarily on the notion that living organisms will do what is necessary to struggle to survive. In this struggle, certain behaviors develop that are defined as "coping mechanisms." "By coping we refer to the things that people do to avoid being harmed by life strains" is the definition offered by Pearlin and Schooler (1978, p. 2). These authors go on to say:

> The protective function of coping behavior can be exercised in three ways: by eliminating or modifying conditions that give rise to problems; by perceptually controlling the meaning of experience in a manner that neutralizes its problematic character; and by keeping the emotional consequences of problems within manageable bounds. (1987, p. 2)

Within these categories, responses that modify the situation are viewed as the most direct way of coping. However, where there is little possibility of changing or eliminating the problem, the stressful impact may be buffered by responses that function to control the meaning of the problem.

In this connection, the conceptual model of Lazarus (1966) and Lazarus and Folkman (1984) is of primary interest. Essentially, this model suggests that it is the *appraisal* of the experience as threatening or innocuous that creates the framework for coping responses. This appraisal also determines whether the experience will continue to be perceived as a stressor or whether it can be neutralized. As the critical mediating variable, appraisal involves three processes: "primary appraisal," or the perception of threat; "secondary appraisal," which involves developing a response to the threat; and "coping," or executing the response. The selection of coping strategies appears to be contingent on the meanings assigned to the problem situation.

Attributional Aspects

Attribution theory deals with how people make sense of their experiences and assign significance to them. It is a process of causal inference, and in the case of schizophrenia, it involves the attempts of victims and their families to make sense out of what is happening to them. We have previously discussed some attributional aspects of symptoms themselves—how a person experiencing paranoid ideation, for example, makes sense out of the triggering impulse by seeing other people as threatening and acting on this perception. This is a temporary, maladaptive attribution in response to an internal stressor.

Few people remain in acute delusional or paranoid states for long periods of time, however. In the long term, most patients become stabilized but still retain their identity as persons with schizophrenia. It is under long-term conditions that attributional processes become particularly important, because persons with schizophrenia have to come to terms with a new definition of who they are, where they fit into society, and what their potential is for a productive life.

Mechanic (1984) has pointed out that when there are changes in physical functioning and feeling states, people tend to test various hypotheses about the seriousness of the symptoms and possible causes, and the manner in which these attributions are made affects the type of actions pursued. With respect to mental disorder, he is interested in

> how people come to attribute causality to their experiences, and more specifically, the locus of causality. Under what conditions, for example, do people come to view their feelings or behavior as a consequence of a moral failure or as a consequence of an illness for which they are not responsible? Particularly in cases where definitions of mental disorder are imposed on individuals by other members of their social group, decisions must be made as to the extent to which the behavior or attitude of the patient reflects "badness" in contrast to "sickness," and these attributions are very much affected by the sociocultural context. (p. 450)

Mechanic goes on the note that attributions of causality affect the care provided, the course of the disorder, and programs of rehabilitation for the patient.

The issue Mechanic describes is one that has commonly been represented as the "madness–badness" dichotomy. When society views certain deviant behaviors in a person, are these attributed to a condition over which he or she has no control, or to an inherent character deficit for which the individual should be punished? This dichotomy underlies the whole issue of accountability and culpability in law. The attribution of madness and badness is a two-pronged issue, however. On one level, society excuses the persons who is "mad" and criminalizes the person who is "bad." This suggests that there is a clear evaluative distinction between the two conditions. The essential question, however, is how the mentally ill individual evaluates his or her own condition. Does the person who has been labeled "mad" also experience himself or herself as "bad"? In terms of attributions, labeling theory suggests that mental illness is experienced as a negative condition only to the extent that society labels it as such.

On another, interrelated level, does the person who is labeled "mad" also experience himself or herself as "sick"? Cultural attributions of madness, badness, and sickness are believed to underlie the prognosis and chronicity of major psychiatric disorders (Lefley, 1990). This may be so because cultural belief systems answer these essential questions for the individual. Many commentators (Estroff, 1981; Harding, Zubin, & Strauss, 1987; Mechanic, 1984) have suggested that if societies treat mentally ill persons as having a serious chronic disability, then they will assume the sick role. Waxler (1984) has proposed that prognosis is better in certain traditional cultures, because these cultures believe that psychiatric disorders are temporary and easily curable aberrations that can happen to anyone. The sick person is not held responsible for the illness; his or her "self" remains unchanged; and it is expected that the symptoms will disappear and the person will quickly return to normal. This is a "normalizing" process that is assumed to result in briefer periods of disability and better long-term prognosis.

The basic underlying concept here is that societal attitudes and expectations are embodied in the coping capabilities of the afflicted individuals. They can get well quickly because society expects them to. Above all, they are not diminished because of their psychiatric disorder in the eyes of society, and therefore they are not diminished in their own self-evaluation. And because of this, the argument goes, such individuals do not stay disordered long enough to assume the identity of disabled persons. Research in developing countries, however, suggests that only some people with schizophrenia respond in this way. At least one-third seem to suffer from intractable conditions, regardless of the cultural context (Lin & Kleinman, 1988; Westermeyer, 1989).

Conceptions of the Self
and Coping Capabilities

Schizophrenia is quintessentially a disturbance of the self. Because concepts and perceptions of the self are deeply embedded in culture, this phenomenon must be regarded from at least two vantage points. First is the personal, phenomenological experience of self-fragmentation and the symbolic meaning of this process. The other is the individual's perception of the self as a discrete entity, a separate human being, surrounded by other members of the culture. The first instance involves self–self boundaries related to personal space and mind–body unity. The second instance involves self–other boundaries, in which both self-as-subject and self-as-object are determined by social context.

There is considerable anthropological evidence that the concept of the person varies cross-culturally (Shweder & Bourne, 1982). Western individualistic cultures tend to view persons as singular entities who can be described in terms of specific personality characteristics that tend to be stable over time. Sociocentric or group-oriented cultures, by contrast, conceptualize "the person" primarily in contextual terms. A person is described in terms of social role and behavior, rather than in terms of qualities that adhere to the self.

The experience of psychosis is a loss of control over one's boundaries and one's prior experienced reality that is essentially terrifying in Western culture. In non-Western or traditional cultures, a change in self or body boundaries such as a trance state may be valued in a ritual context, but in a nonritual context it is likely to be perceived as mental disorder, the same as in the West (Lefley, 1984). Torrey (1988) describes the "inner world of madness" as a fearful state involving alteration of the senses; inability to synthesize, sort, or integrate stimuli; feelings of unreality; and an altered sense of self, including detachment of one's body. Frightening delusions or hallucinations accompany the experience. These have been described in even greater detail by writers who have suffered schizophrenia and recall the altered sense of self and the "me–not me" differentiation (Kytle, 1987; North, 1987).

As noted in Chapter 1, Estroff (1989) describes schizophrenia as "an *I am* illness—one that may overtake and redefine the identity of the person" (p. 189). Estroff notes that there are two conflicting conceptions of schizophrenia in relation to self in the Western world: (1) Loss of self *is* the illness ("there is no formed or cohering self in schizophrenia," p. 193); and (2) the illness experience results in a loss of and change in self. The first view is described more precisely by Fabrega (1989): "The schizophrenia lesion or vulnerability factor is held à la Kraepelin and Bleuler to affect deleteriously the integration of affect, will, volition, and cognition that gives the person a sense of unity" (p. 278). In Estroff's view, the first definition informs the second; the professional definition of schizophrenia defeats the person with schizophrenia, leading to a loss of self and positive social roles, and thus to chronicity. Fabrega (1989), however, suggests that the patient's acceptance of his or her culture's definition of the self is what leads to a fused identity with the illness:

> The Western self that underpins biomedical notions about health and illness is assumed to be autonomous, free, and in control. In eroding its symbolic organization, schizophrenia alters the self's sense of wholeness, integration, and the cultural boundaries that give it coherence, an outcome of this being feelings of passivity, lack of control, social alienation, etc. (p. 281)

COPING STRATEGIES IN SCHIZOPHRENIA

Lazarus and Folkman (1984), in their Ways of Coping Scale, have differentiated between two major types of coping. "Problem-focused" coping is aimed at resolving the problem or taking action to eliminate or change the source of stress. "Emotion-focused" coping is oriented toward managing the emotional distress evoked by the stressful situation. Carver, Scheier, and Weintraub (1989) have discovered conceptually distinct aspects of problem-focused coping, including active coping or direct action; planning; and seeking instrumental social support, such as advice, assistance, and information. Emotion-focused coping also has discrete factors: seeking emotional social support, such as sympathy and understanding; positive reinterpretation (reappraising a distressful event as a learning or growth experience; acceptance of the reality of the situation; turning to religion; and "denial" or a reappraisal of the seriousness of the stressor, which is sometimes protective. An interesting insight by Mechanic (1984) also suggests that a coping mechanism that might otherwise be labeled as "denial" may be helpful in coming to terms with the unusual changes in the life of a person with a major mental disorder. In some instances symptomatic behavior is "normalized and the person does not become a patient" (p. 451). There are also coping resources that are less useful and that may be maladaptive: a focus on emotional issues and ventilation of affect, and behavioral or mental disengagement. These strategies avoid acknowledging and dealing with the problem.

Problem-focused coping is generally operative when people feel that it is within their power to control or deal constructively with a stressor. Emotion-focused coping tends to be the response when people feel that a stressor is too difficult to manage, control, or overcome. In terms of face validity, problem-focused coping seems to be more adaptive than emotion-focused coping. For persons with schizophrenia, however, active planning and actions to deal with the multiple stressors of the disease and its sequelae have been impeded by an indifferent world and even by overprotective service providers (Estroff, 1981). In point of fact, for persons who are disabled by schizophrenic symptoms, active coping is generally possible only under certain conditions. For many, the family or service provider system offers the medium for planning and instrumental support. Patients' willingness to avail themselves of that which is offered — rehabilitation, skill building, resocialization, and medication for symptom stabilization — may be considered under the rubric of active coping. It is only in recent years that patients have taken matters into their own hands by developing consumer advocacy organizations and consumer-operated services. In the main, coping strategies have tended to be emotion-focused. Much of this coping response derives from an appraisal of the service delivery system as a stressor, and of patients as impotent pawns in the hands of others.

Why is appraisal so critical in schizophrenia? It is this single variable, we believe, that mediates for the afflicted person the meaning and evaluation of the symptomatic condition. Appraisal is the processing of the stressful event and the actions one must take to deal with it. In schizophrenia, this involves an array of defenses used to develop an explanatory model of the psychotic episode, the treatment by others, and the subsequent changes in one's life.

Persons who have experienced psychotic episodes may respond with denial, anger, shame, or reassessment of self, to name just a few of a large repertoire of defenses. When the person perceives her or his own behavior as normal whereas others in the culture have judged it abnormal, we may assume that this denial is a function of the state of the illness. But once a person is stabilized, and is able to acknowledge that she or he is indeed mentally ill, the defenses involved in appraisal of that identification may focus on the self or on others. Shame, self-devaluation, and feelings of being diminished are intropunitive responses that focus on the self. Anger at incarceration and disempowerment focus on others. Although persons with schizophrenia write often and profoundly about the terrors of psychosis, for many former patients appraisal of the experience of mental illness remains fixated on the humiliating external events surrounding the psychotic episode. Thus, over and over again at gatherings with former patients, we hear their outrage at being held against their will, stripped of power and control of their own bodies, and forced to submit to the judgment of others regarding their own fate.

Anger at the System as a Coping Response

In our culture, the recollections of persons with mental illness are frequently characterized by one overriding emotion: anger. The self-selected identifications of consumer groups as "inmates" or "survivors"; the choice of the term "ex-mental patient" rather than the euphemistic "client"; and the antipsychiatry stance of many of the ex-patient groups give open evidence of their antipathy to the professionals who believe they have helped them (Emerick, 1990). The consumer movement, indeed, has been divided by the degree rather than the quality of an anger that seems to be widely prevalent but is targeted toward different goals. For some consumers, anger fuels total rejection of the mental health system; for others, it lubricates their efforts to make the system more responsive to their needs.

Why is there this ubiquitous anger, and what is its basis? It is not even necessary to do content analysis to see the patterns that are in bold relief in every account: humiliation, failure to be listened to or understood, and overwhelming powerlessness are the three unifying themes. It is clear that in Western culture, at any rate, current and former mental patients have had more negative than positive experiences with the healing system. As a group, they feel abused, aggressed against, mistreated. What they remember are restraints, involuntary incarceration, sometimes medications administered against their will, and frequently psychological abuse from professionals viewed as indifferent or punitive (Chamberlin, 1978). There are indeed some positive memories, but when good things are mentioned, they are often described in terms of contrast. Professionals help when they do the opposite of what the bad professionals have done: when they trust, reinforce autonomy, remove constraints, and give space (Leete, 1987b). Good professionals are typically those who undo damage, whether it is societal, familial, or iatrogenic.

For a long time, then, a major coping strategy of persons with long-term schizophrenia—particularly those who have a history of hospitalization—has been emotion-focused ventilation. The stressor, the perceived threat, has not been the illness itself, but rather the system that purportedly serves those with the illness. Although some former mental patients have used behavioral and mental disengagement, many have banded together in organized groups with the avowed purpose of active coping through changing the service delivery system. In this endeavor, an emphasis on independence and consumer empowerment has become a major coping strategy. This emphasis is directed toward relations with professionals, but it also redresses the poor self-image and powerlessness that have been salient features of the illness itself. An important feature of this coping response has been the movement toward providing consumer-developed and consumer-operated services for peers, on the premise that experience conveys expertise and no one understands the problems better than those who have been afflicted by mental illness.

A recent study of 104 self-help groups for former mental patients by Emerick (1990) suggests that we may now be entering a new developmental stage of active coping by persons with a schizophrenic illness. Emerick has identified two major service models among these groups. The "social movement" model is oriented toward social change and offers services such as legal advocacy, public education, technical assistance, and information–referral networking. "In contrast, the individual therapy groups provide their members with opportunities for more 'inner-focused' individual change through group support meetings, drop-in centers, and various types of 'alternative therapy' " (p. 402). If we apply the factors indicated by Carver et al. (1989), the strategies now in evidence include active coping and planning, as well as seeking and obtaining instrumental and emotional social support.

Within these two service models are three categories of group structure describing relations with mental health professionals. "Separatist" groups do not allow professionals to be members; "supportive" groups permit professionals to participate in auxiliary roles, and "partnership" groups allow professionals to act as leaders in partnership with members who are former patients. Among these groups, 62.5% are social movement groups and 37.5% are individual therapy groups. In the social movement category, 20% are separatist, 58% are supportive, and 22% are partnership groups. In the individual therapy category, 10% are separatist, 69% are supportive, and 21% are partnership groups. Overall, 16% are separatist, 63% are supportive, and 21% are partnership groups.

Although professional participation is obviously permitted to a large extent in these groups, and most report some interaction with professionals, the degree of interaction is very low. Professionals do not seem to avail themselves of their rights to participate. More than 70% of the groups report no to low interaction with professionals, as opposed to fewer than 30% reporting moderate to high interaction. Most telling is the attitudinal response. The largest proportion of groups in the sample (42.8%) held antiprofessional attitudes, while only 26.2% had favorable attitudes toward professionals and 30.9% were neutral. Therapy groups tend to be more amenable to professional alliances, and social movement groups more antagonistic; this is predictable, given the development of many social movement groups on an antipsychiatry platform. Nevertheless, Emerick concludes that the fact that most groups are involved in at least some interaction bodes well for the future of professional partnerships. He cites the first national symposium of self-help groups and providers in March 1989 in Chicago, which "may well result in a tempering both of strong antiprofessional sentiments in patient groups and of antiself-help attitudes among professionals" (1990, p. 406).

Continuing Questions about Coping with Schizophrenia

In developing coping strengths, persons with schizophrenia are faced with formidable challenges; some are intrinsic to the disease process, and others are extrinsic, involving dealing with questions of identification as mentally ill persons and the attendant social stigma. In this process, some basic definitional aspects become blurred. Whether the individual defines schizophrenia as a disease to be accepted and overcome to the greatest extent possible, or whether schizophrenia is defined as a social label to be denied through political efforts, determines the coping strategies that will be developed to deal with the disorder.

In this chapter we have suggested that identification of a person as being schizophrenic, or as having schizophrenia, is dependent on both cultural definition of and cultural responses to mental illness, and that many of the coping strategies developed are responsive to these parameters. What of the definitions assigned by the mental health establishment? Although many elements of the service delivery system are viewed as reinforcing the sick role (Estroff, 1981; Harding, Zubin, & Strauss, 1987), over at least the past quarter century professionals have followed a pattern of demedicalizing mental illness. The term "client" has been substituted for "patient"; the terms "serious and persistent" have been substituted for "chronic," a neutral medical concept applied to diseases such as diabetes, which can be stabilized but for which there are no known cures. Bachrach (1986) is opposed to these semantic strategies and to the thinking behind them. She has noted that the British now have terms for three kinds of chronic patients: "old long-stay," "new long-stay," and "short-stay." Moreover, she points out that substituting "client" for "patient" may be maladaptive for the very persons this redefinition purports to help. She agrees with those who feel "that people who are sick already have enough to deal with, without expending energy on seeking their own boundaries" (p. 31), and that until the "patient" identity is accepted there is difficulty in mobilizing coping strengths for more productive endeavors. It should also be pointed out that continuing to view such words as stigmatizing reinforces the stigma of the referent.

Is it possible to accept a "patient" identity and at the same time to eschew the dependency and sick role that are so often associated with that label? There are persons who recognize the boundaries imposed by their illness and who are articulate about the strategies they use to structure their time, bolster their self-concept, improve socialization experiences, and avoid excessive environmental stimulation or distraction. Esso Leete (1989) had given us a careful description of such coping mechanisms, evolving from long experience. This requires a recognition of schizophrenia as a mental disorder and acknowledgment of its handicapping features. At the same time, Leete and many others like her are involved in organizational advocacy efforts to overcome stigma, prejudice, and discrimination against persons with mental illnesses. This combination of individual and social strategies seems to be the very essence of problem-focused active coping. In forthcoming chapters, we describe the paradigms used by other people in adapting to the realities of living with schizophrenic illness.

SUMMARY AND CONCLUSIONS

In this chapter we have used schizophrenia as an example of biologically based long-term mental illnesses that traditionally have been interpreted in a psychodynamic idiom. In contrast, we view schizophrenia and similar disorders as disease processes with special personal and social meanings that affect psychological response.

Using a model of stress, coping, and adaptation, the chapter has been concerned with the self-perception of persons with schizophrenia in relation to the immediate and larger social environment. We have suggested that both internal and external stimuli may trigger a series of responses that seem to be based on a certain maladaptive inner logic. The trajectory of events may begin with neurotransmitter dysfunctions that lead to misinterpretations of social stimuli as threatening or hostile. The person's subsequent aberrant behavior may then evoke a negative social response that reinforces the original misinterpretation. In this model the symptomatic behaviors represent coping responses to perceived threat rather than psychodynamic metaphors for unresolved conflicts. To understand schizophrenia as a biopsychosocial phenomenon, it is suggested that social psychological theories of stress and coping, attribution, and self-concept, as well as life events research, are relevant to the intensity and course of illness.

Coping and adaption theory becomes the framework for analyzing schizophrenic behavior. Attribution theory also provides a backdrop for analyzing how people with schizophrenia make sense out of their own cognitive perceptions and feeling states and how they internally process other people's reactions to their behavior. The major issue relates to long-term self-attribution. Do individuals with a stabilized mental illness internalize society's negative views, label themselves as defective, and adopt a disabled role? Cultural attributions of madness, badness, and sickness are believed to have a part in the prognosis and chronicity of major psychiatric disorders. Similarly, cultural conceptions of the self may affect whether a person's identity becomes fused with her or his illness.

Coping strategies of persons with schizophrenia and other major psychiatric disorders may range from denial to acceptance, from emotional ventilation and diffuse anger at the system to highly focused organization, advocacy, and development of alternative services. We suggest that optimal coping is exemplified by persons who acknowledge their psychiatric disability and who make every effort to overcome its handicapping features. These are people who utilize treatment effectively and who often derive insights from the experiences. Effective coping strategies also involve participation in advocacy efforts to overcome societal stigma and discrimination against people with mental illness.

HOW PATIENTS EXPERIENCE PSYCHOSIS

CHAPTER THREE

Disturbances in the Sense of Self

The next three chapters concern themselves with the way men and women with schizophrenia and other major mental illnesses experience psychosis. It is clear from the personal accounts that follow that many individuals suffer a substantial transformation of their personal world in the course of mental illness. In most of the accounts we do not know the individual's particular diagnosis. We can only judge from the experiences they share that they have undergone profound psychotic experiences. According to DSM-III-R (American Psychiatric Association, 1987), psychotic disturbances may be found in schizophrenia, paranoid disorder, major depression, manic episodes, and other disorders. It is difficult to say at this time how psychotic experiences may differ among diagnostic categories. Because most of the literature about psychosis occurs in the context of schizophrenia, we have necessarily emphasized that diagnostic category more heavily in this section.

The subject matter of the next three chapters focuses on the major disturbances that occur in the psychotic experience — disturbances in the sense of self, in cognition, emotions, relationships, and behaviors. The present chapter introduces the discussion with attention to disturbances in the sense of self, which are probably more prevalent in schizophrenia than in other major mental disorders.

DISTURBED PERCEPTION AS A PRIMARY FACTOR

A disturbed sense of self may involve a sense of loss of ego boundaries, an extreme perplexity about one's identity, or specific delusions about being controlled by outside forces. Although these changes are in many ways individual, there are common threads that make it possible to discuss them. Drawing from his work on schizophrenia, Corbett (1976) argues that disturbed perceptions are primary in psychosis because they (1) occur first, (2) are the point of departure for other manifestations of the disease, (3) are psychologically irreducible, and (4) are the closest psychological events to the original pathological process. This leads Corbett to consider schizophrenia to be a "perceptual dyscontrol syndrome" (p. 251). He leans heavily on the work of Merleau-Ponty for his argument that perception is primary, that "the world is what we perceive" (Corbett, 1976, p. 251), and that perception is the background against which all actions occur.

Men and women suffering from psychosis experience a wide range of perceptual distortions. The perceptual world may be flooded with images that they cannot control. They may experience significant changes in intensity of stimuli; things may look strange and unreal; and objects may change in size and shape. There may be abnormal time and space perceptions, distortions of bodily sensations, and changes in the perception of emotions (Corbett, 1976; Torrey, 1983, 1988).

Persons with psychosis suffer from high levels of stress and anxiety as they strive to negotiate the world of their inner experience and the world they share with others. When their perceptions go awry, they lose the sense of environmental stability that would allow them to function with comfort and confidence. They lack the capacity to organize perceptions to manageable proportions. Antonovsky (1979), who studied factors that affect human health and well-being, has concluded that the irreducible element in well-being is a "sense of coherence," which he defines as "an enduring though dynamic feeling of confidence that one's internal and external environment are predictable and that things will work out as well as can be expected" (p. 123). The lack of coherence and predictability plagues the lives of those with major mental illnesses, and often overwhelms their capacities to cope.

THE LOSS OF A SENSE OF SELF

As indicated in the last chapter, the experience of psychosis, with its loss of ego boundaries and sense of unreality, can be terrifying—especially in Western culture. Again, Estroff (1989) sees the loss of sense of self as central to schizophrenia and therefore suggests that it might best be called an "I am" illness—an illness that tends to encompass the identity of the person. Although, as we will see later in this chapter, this may not be a fully adequate conceptualization of all psychotic disorders, many of the following quotations seem to support the idea that many patients in some stages of their illness *are* their illness.

For example, Mary Louise Sharp (1987) says about her psychotic experience:

> It's hard to describe what real psychosis is because when you are in it, it's hard to be clear. The world seems under water, and my nervous system on the outside, buffeted by mental winds, blinking lights and dog barks that might as well be guns and tanks from my pain and despair. (p. 1)

Mary McGrath (1984), whose first-person account is titled "Where Did I Go?," reveals herself puzzling about her reflection in a store window and asking, "It's me, isn't it?" She says, "I know it is, but it's hard to tell" (p. 638). She knows that she is a sculptor and a writer, but still her identity seems to her undefined. McGrath values the help of a therapist in her fearful times, for "She listens when I need to release some of the 'poisons' in my mind. . . . She sees me as a human being and not only a body to shovel pills into or a cerebral mass in some laboratory" (p. 639).

Landis and Mettler (1964) collected first-person accounts of serious mental illness and found that many of their informants talked about feeling fundamentally separated from the world that other people inhabit, feeling themselves to be in limbo, or feeling like walking ghosts. The authors quoted one patient as saying:

> It was just that sometimes I had a terrific sense of unreality. Suddenly I found myself in the present and all the immediate cords to the present had been severed. Like when someone wakes up in a strange room. Except that I had lived in the room for months. . . . I often felt dazed. (Landis & Mettler, 1964, p. 361)

Some patients report that they have felt different from others since childhood. Cathy King-Hasher (1989) found other children acting and reacting to each other spontaneously in a way that she was never able to fathom:

> Myself, I felt inundated by all the details of every interaction and had to sort them out consciously to determine how I should act and what I should do in even the simplest situations, such as another child taking my toy, or the teacher asking me how many brothers and sisters I had. As I stood stiffly, overwhelmed, trying to piece it all together, the time to act has passed. Everyone seemed to be part of a movie and I could not find my way in it. (p. 8)

In her great perplexity, King-Hasher suddenly arrived at the notion that she was neither boy nor girl, but someone in between. "I am

not one of those people at all," she decided. "I'm of a different species. That's why people are all against me" (p. 8). Now she sees this
as a standard paranoid delusion: "They are all against me because I
am special" (p. 8).

Kaplan (1964) includes part of Jane Hillyard's 1926 account of
her mental illness in his collection of first person accounts. Hillyard
described her experience, which Kaplan feels to be suggestive of depression, as follows:

> A feeling of being lost, lost utterly with no sense of place or time,
> no idea as to who voices belonged [to], no clear realization of my
> identity, lost in mind and body and soul, lost to light and form and
> color: a distinct, acid nausea of self-revulsion—all of these were
> in the feeling that swept over me. (Kaplan, 1964, p. 160)

"If I want to reach out to touch me, I feel nothing but slippery
coldness," McGrath (1984) writes, "yet I sense it is me." Later in the
article she says, "My existence seems undefined—[a] mere image that
I keep reaching for, but can never touch" (p. 638).

The difficulty of intervening in the strange world of the mentally
ill is experienced by clinicians and families alike. Nona Borgeson (1982)
provides a possible explanation:

> Where weighing the odds of probability ends, schizophrenia begins,
> and paranoia runs rampant. The schizophrenic doesn't think; he/she
> knows, false knowledge though it be, and his/her world becomes
> one of polarities—black or white, love or hate, ecstasy, or suicidal
> inclinations, mortal fear or indestructibility. (p. 7)

These first-person accounts of mental illness and the way the self
seems to fragment and disintegrate gives substance to Estroff's asser-
tion that schizophrenia might be considered an "I am" disorder. Further considerable difficulty arises for the individual, Estroff notes, when
the private world comes into conflict with the way the person is seen
by others. When these perceptions do not coincide, the person is certain to experience an overwhelming sense of estrangement and alien-
ation.

Estroff (1989) raises another provocative issue when she begins
asking questions regarding the continuity of the sense of self. When
family members talk about a relative with mental illness, they draw
a sharp contrast between the person they knew before he or she became ill and the radical changes they now witness. But Estroff asks,
"Is the person so different, so altered, so absent, as we have thought?
Is there a missing person associated with schizophrenia or is the per-

son present but obscured from our recognition?" (p. 191). At present, she acknowledges, we do not have the information that would clarify what is the same and what is different when schizophrenia occurs. We need to study the processes and experiences of change, loss, and persistence of self accompanying schizophrenia.

The struggle for self goes on both privately and publicly, in terms of the inner sense of self and in terms of social identity. If this struggle is successful, these men and women may experience the self as persisting, but with some new features or incapacities. What becomes important, then, is the meaning of the illness to the person. This needs to be recognized and acknowledged, and the person needs to be helped to deal with the unique meanings that the experience of mental illness has for him or her.

ALTERED SENSE OF SELF

In the preceding section we have presented examples of psychotic experiences in which people suffer a sense of loss of self. In this section we provide examples of experiences characterized by distortions in perceptions of the body and those in which new identities are assumed.

Torrey (1983) has identified cases in which various body parts of the patient take on a life of their own. A male patient reported the following experience:

> My breast gives the impression of a pretty well-developed female bosom; this phenomenon can be seen by anybody who wants to observe me *with his own eyes*. . . . A brief glance will not suffice. The observer would have to go to the trouble of spending ten or fifteen minutes near me. In that way anybody would notice the periodic swelling and diminution of my bosom. (p. 34; emphasis the patient's)

Torrey found other schizophrenic patients who confused their identities with those of others. For example, one patient related this experience:

> I was myself in different bodies. . . .The night nurse came in and sat under the shaded lamp in a quiet ward. I recognized her as me, and I watched for some time quite fascinated; I had never had an outside view of myself before. In the morning several of the patients having breakfast were me. I recognized them by the way they held their knives and forks. (p. 34)

Some patients take on the identity of a highly desirable character whom all can emulate. Frederick J. Frese (Chapter 6, this volume) describes a highly gratifying "cosmic experience," in which he became "Uncle Fred" to his friends and later to the patients in the hospital to which he was committed.

Many patients who have provided personal accounts have taken on identities with highly grandiose dimensions. David Zelt (1989) reports such an experience, describing himself in the third person:

> During the next few weeks, David came to believe that he was the reborn figure of Jesus Christ and that their spirits were identical. Like Christ, he was constantly in touch with the infinite and the eternal, and lived with a halo around his head that represented unity with God. (p. 45)

A heightened sense of awareness predominates in some phases of some psychosis. Judy Doughty (1987) remembers finding feathers everywhere and believing that they were a special sign of something wonderful to come. The air was fresher and cleaner than she had ever known. She had a strong sensation that something momentous was about to happen.

Some clinicians have expressed concern that the gratification in these kinds of experiences may result in resistance to recovery (Mac-Kinnon, 1977; McGlashan & Carpenter, 1976). A patient's sense of individuality and personal identity may reside largely in the psychotic experience and may be difficult to give up. Such ambivalence about schizophrenia is found in McGrath's (1984) account:

> Should I let anyone know that there are moments, just moments in schizophrenia that are "special"? When I feel I am traveling to someplace I can't go "normally"? Where there is an awareness, a different sort of vision allowed me? Moments which I can't make myself believe are just symptoms of craziness and nothing more . . . the times when colors appear brighter, alluring almost, and my attention is drawn into the shadows, the lights, the intricate patterns of texture, the bold outlines of objects around me . . . and everything is wonder. (p. 63)

MacKinnon (1977) presents excerpts from a patient's letter that illustrates the intensity, sense of purpose, and feeling of personal significance that psychosis brought to one man's life. Even though some of his experiences were fraught with fear, they were more rewarding than ordinary everyday experiences, which can have their personal failures and humiliations. The patient wrote:

> I really missed my illness when I was free of it. I guess what I missed
> most was the sense of mystery. My visual hallucinations filled me
> with wonder and awe, as well as scaring me more than any horror
> movie ever could have done. When I turned the Bible to the first
> page and found that the wording had all changed, it sent shivers
> up and down my spine. The first hallucination I had was really
> frightening. My brother-in-law was smiling at me when suddenly
> his features blurred and I saw the devil staring back at me. (p. 427)

The personal significance of psychotic experience can be seen
repeatedly in patient's accounts of their illness. Even when the delusions are persecutory, some people see them as meaningful. As one
of MacKinnon's subjects explained about a bad experience, its importance for him lay in the belief that God thought he was so special that
He was punishing him like this. He said he felt quite let down to find
that his religious experience "was all fraud and that people weren't
really writing songs and magazine article about me" (MacKinnon, 1977,
p. 427).

One individual who had a particularly gratifying experience found
that this experience was helpful to her in her recovery:

> My first psychotic episode appeared as a private mental exorcism,
> ending with the honor of sainthood and gifts of hope and faith.
> Fortunately, this sense of power became a source of tremendous
> strength during my recovery and sustains me even today. (Hough-
> ton, 1982, p. 549)

DISORDERS OF ATTENTION

Patients' statement about the experience of mental illness frequently
reveal deficits in attentional focus. Freedman (1974), who studied over
50 autobiographical books and articles written by patients, noted that
over half of them reported problems in concentrating on reading, writing, and speaking, or said that their minds wandered a great deal. A
patient quoted by Torrey (1983) provides the following example:

> My concentration is poor. I jump from one thing to another. If I
> am talking to someone, they only need to cross their legs or scratch
> their heads and I am distracted and forget what I am saying. I think
> I could concentrate better with my eyes shut. (p. 10)

One explanation for this dilemma lies in the difficulty these people have in filtering out irrelevant detail and controlling that to which
they will attend (Freedman, 1974; McGhie & Chapman, 1961; Tor-

rey, 1983). It is as if the brain is being flooded with both internal and external stimuli. McGhie and Chapman reported such examples as "I let all sounds come in that are there" or "There are too many things coming into my head at once" (1961, p. 105). Ordinarily people are able to filter out unwanted stimuli and to attend selectively to that which is relevant, but people with schizophrenia seem to be deficient in these protective buffering mechanism. The irrelevant seems to have as much salience for them as the relevant. Some patients have reported that their inability to concentrate was impaired by the intrusion of hallucinatory material (Freedman, 1974).

Anscombe (1987) makes a strong case for the argument that an attentional deficit is primary in schizophrenia and that most other symptoms of the disorder follow from it. He supports this view by noting that many patients report a sensation of being captured by a stimulus rather than being able to choose what to attend to. Minor factors (e.g., colors, textures, or blemishes) attract these persons with a salience out of proportion to their importance. Patients cannot shift their attention flexibly, not because of its importance, but because they lack the capacity for control.

Attention may jam so that a person remains stuck for minutes on end. In the following example, the person is blocked by something of little consequence:

> If I am reading I may suddenly get bogged down at a word. It may be any word, even a simple word that I know well. When this happens I cannot get past it. It is as if I am being hypnotized by it. It's as if I am seeing it for the first time and in a different way from anyone else. It's not so much that I absorb it, it's more like it is absorbing me. (Patient quoted in McGhie & Chapman, 1961, p. 109)

With objects appearing to jump out and command attention, it is understandable that people with schizophrenia feel that these objects to which they are so powerfully attracted have great importance for them. Things appear significant because they have captured attention, and the persons feel impelled to make sense of it in some way. David Zelt (1989), again telling his story in the third person, illustrates the point:

> Ordinarily unimportant information from external reality took on new dimensions for him. For example, colors powerfully influenced him. At any moment wherever David went, colors were used to express judgments about his spirituality. People used the colors of the clothes or cars to express positive or negative views of him. Green

meant that David was like Christ; white stood for his spiritual purity; orange indicated he was attuned to the cosmos. (p. 48)

Anscombe (1987) says that the person's lack of control over attention makes for passivity. Unable to choose a focus, the person becomes the audience of his or her mental life, rather than its initiator. This, Anscombe believes, is a prime factor in the loss of the sense of self or the role of the "I" as the agent in his or her own life. There follows the loss of identity and with it a loss of kinship with other people.

Some patients give up the struggle to assert themselves and undergo experiences that hardly seem to be their own:

> Things just happen to me now and I have no control over them. I don't seem to have the same say in things anymore. At times, I can't even control what I want to think about. I am starting to feel pretty numb about everything because I am becoming an object and objects don't have feelings. (Patient quoted in McGhie & Chapman, 1961, p. 109)

> The most sacred monument that is erected by the human spirit, i.e. its ability to think and decide and will to do, is torn apart by itself. . . . things . . . are done by something that seems mechanical and frightening because it is able to do things and unable to want to or not want to. (Meyer & Covi, 1960, quoted in Anscombe, 1987, p. 255)

The capturing of attention and the apparent role of external circumstances in assigning meanings lead to a variety of interpretations— telepathy, thought control, and electronic brain implants. Unable to direct their attention to other experiences or data from long-term memory, which might help them correct and reassess impressions, these people yield to delusional thinking.

PERSON-DISORDER INTERACTIONS

The patient perceptions presented thus far in this chapter might lead us to conclude that schizophrenia is indeed an "I am" phenomenon (Estroff, 1989). People do seem to "be" their illnesses. They seem to have lost their sense of self, or the self has been so altered that another person seems to have taken over. Volition, self-control, and will power have disappeared. The persons seem to have lost control of their lives and to be at the mercy of internal and external forces.

Examination of accounts given by other patients or by the same patients in another phase of the illness, however, often reveals a significantly different picture—one in which the persons are actively seeking control of symptoms and making decisions about life. For example, John J. Cunningham, a patient interviewed by Irvine (1985), arrived rather suddenly at an awareness that he could be an active agent in his own recovery. He came to this realization after suffering the most serious relapse of his life:

> I was on my back and it was like waking from a bad dream, if you will pardon a very tired analogy. But that's what it was like. I was frightened. Now I knew that it wasn't anyone else's fault, that it was no one else's job, it was mine. I had the power if I wanted to, to become a person who goes to work in the morning, or sits in the park and doesn't have to be sick. . . . it was "readiness" and disposition and good luck. (Irvine, 1985, p. 76)

Esso Leete has written and spoken extensively about her experience with mental illness. She says that contrary to popular thinking that people with schizophrenia are withdrawn and passive, they are actively fighting "internal terrors and external realities" to keep their emotional balance and social composure in a world they cannot always translate. She has made a conscious decision to learn to understand the illness and to manage it in such a way that it does not control her life. She believes that doing these things is up to the individual and that they can be done (Leete, 1987a, 1987b). The language in her chapter in this book (see Chapter 10) indicates the great extent to which she has become an active agent in her own recovery: "I have become an expert in my illness"; "I have absorbed my losses and been surprised at my victories"; "I have learned coping mechanisms." This strong sense of personal control emerges throughout the chapter, even though for many years Leete and her family were not given much hope.

Jeannette Keil (1984) found that she could learn to control her words and actions even if she was unable to control her racing thoughts. She worked persistently to keep her life in balance, and she pressured herself to appear appropriate. Another patient, Barbara Bair-Nichols, was motivated to do something about her life because she so much hated being physically restrained in the hospital. She said that was the basis of her recovery (Savelson, 1986).

Strauss has written extensively in the past decades about the psychological side of schizophrenia; he has persistently sought to learn the extent to which patients are inevitable victims of their illness and the extent to which they can have an impact on their own situation (Strauss, 1987, 1989a; Strauss, Harding, Hafez, & Lieberman, 1987;

Brier & Strauss, 1983). The various attributions of causality in schizophrenia through the ages, such as devil theories, lack of moral fiber, and inadequate coping skills, have invariably affected the way in which afflicted persons regard themselves. These models of mental illness, plus more recent ones of "bad families" and organic causation, leave people with the idea that they can have no impact on their own situation. They are helpless in the face of their environment or their biology. Yet extensive studies of patients' accounts of coping with mental illness reveal that they do feel they can influence their situation (Strauss et al., 1987).

Strauss et al. (1987) note that we still lack data about the role that patients play in their own recovery. In fact, we lack conceptual models and exploratory research in the area. On the basis of many patients' autobiographical accounts, the authors suggest that people interact with their disorders in various ways and that it is useful to think of three levels or phases of development:

1. The first level is that of compliance with treatment. Although this appears to be a fairly passive role for a person, it does involve willingness on his or her part to accept the treatment offered. The patient can and does choose whether or not to comply.

2. The second level is that of utilizing coping skills training. This kind of training is often done in a complaint frame of mind. People go through the exercises predetermined by the rehabilitation counselor. Still, they probably learn skills that enable them to make more choices and have more control over their lives.

3. On the third level, a patient is actively engaged and serves as collaborator and innovator in his or her own recovery. Courage and hope are important on this level, as is the construction of meaning that the person gives to his or her illness. The person becomes active in figuring out how to manage his or her own symptoms and how to deal with residual impairments.

In a recent article, Strauss (1989b) has made clear that he does not feel that the person and the disorder are the same. We need to think much more about the person who has the disorder and about how he or she interacts with the illness. In particular, we need to give more attention to the feelings, interpretations, and actions that influence the course of the disorder. In Strauss's experience, patients consciously or unconsciously appear to adjust their perceptions, interpretations, and actions to maintain a level of self-esteem; they remain on plateaus of development in order to recuperate; and they use footholds in one aspect of life before taking another step. Clinicians need to observe these coping behaviors and give support to patients as they struggle for self-direction.

We cannot explain very well at this time the psychological factors that influence improvement in functioning and what biological and environmental factors may be operating in conjunction with these. One interesting explanation is that people's attributions or casual explanations, including those pertaining to degree of control (controllable vs. uncontrollable), locus of control (internal vs. external), and degree of stability (stable vs. unstable) strongly influence people's attitudes and behaviors (Kelley & Michela, 1980). People with mental illnesses who feel that they can control aspects of their lives in a fairly predictable way tend to function better. People who believe that internal and external factors control them, by contrast, experience an absence of efficacy, powerlessness, and fatalism; they feel like pawns in their situation and are less persistent in coping.

SUMMARY

Patients' accounts of their experiences with severe mental illnesses reveal that they do indeed suffer a great variety of alterations in sense of self. Some feel that they are being completely engulfed by their illness, and others believe that they have become someone highly different. These things just seem to happen beyond the patients' control, particularly in the acute phases of an illness. In ways we do not understand, greater integration of the self occurs with medications, and in some cases people cycle out of acute psychosis without treatment. It is probable that environment plays a part in the recovery of the self, but we do not know how exactly this occurs.

We need research to demonstrate the relationship between various irregularities of brain functioning and the individual's concept of himself or herself. We need to understand to what extent an inherent healing process may occur and in what ways medications work. We also need to know what caregivers can do to enhance the healing process, even when an individual seems largely tuned out.

What emerges from this discussion is how critical it is in achieving good outcome for these people to begin to feel that they can exert control over their own lives. Basic to coping and adaptation theory is the assumption that there is an inherent predisposition toward adaptive functioning in human beings (Pearlin & Schooler, 1978). Many of the quotations from patients included in this chapter indicate that people do arrive at their own decisions to take charge of their lives and that they figure out for themselves what they can do to manage symptoms and exert control. Once they have arrived at the crucial understanding that they are not powerless—that they can become active agents in their own lives—things become considerably better for them.

It becomes critical, then, that treatment and rehabilitation personnel listen to these persons and their attributions about control. To what extent do these individuals imply that there are aspects of life under their control, and to what extent do they assume that they are victims of internal and external forces? To what extent are their attributions in accord with reality as we best know it? To assume that more can be controlled than is possible at this time can lead to failure and discouragement. Finally, what can caregivers say or do to help these persons shift from a feeling of powerlessness and victimization to one of efficacy and self-direction?

All of us who work with persons with mental illnesses, whether family members, clinicians, or rehabilitation personnel, need to listen to ourselves to determine what messages we are giving about patients' potential for becoming more active agents in their own lives. To what extent are we unwittingly abetting patients in their efforts to assign all negative life circumstances to their disabilities, their families, their peers, or the "system"? On the other hand, to what extent are we telling them it is "all up to them" and letting them suffer one failure after another? We need to observe and listen, in order to make a realistic determination of what can be under their control. Then our language and behavior must clearly and consistently reflect these carefully made assumptions.

CHAPTER FOUR

Disturbances in Cognition

Disturbance in thinking has long been thought to be a primary characteristic of patients with schizophrenia. Bleuler (1911/1950), for example, regarded thought disorder as the most important psychological dysfunction in schizophrenia. For him it was the direct consequence of loosening of associations, which he considered basic to the condition and delusions as an attempt at recovery. The primary problem, he thought, was attributable to brain dysfunction.

According to DSM-III-R (American Psychiatric Association, 1987), people with schizophrenia suffer a disturbance in the content of thought, resulting in delusions that are often fragmented and bizarre. Individuals may be convinced that their thoughts are being broadcast, and that thoughts have been removed from or inserted in their heads. There are also disturbances in forms of thought, such as loosening of associations, poverty of content, or excessive concretism.

Spohn et al. (1986) believe that people with schizophrenic disorders do not experience events as connected; therefore, they have little confidence in the continuity of events. They experience reality as fragmentary, disjointed, and unpredictable. The authors stress the need for research to determine whether thought disorder predates the illness; if so, it might be used as an indicator of vulnerability early in the life of an individual. Spohn et al. also note that the more severe thought disturbances tend to be alleviated by neuroleptics, but that the less severe often persist. Drugs may be selective in terms of the thought patterns they normalize. If residual thought disturbances remain severe, all areas of adjustment are affected, and prognosis is poor.

Recent research has shown that mental illnesses other than schizophrenia may also be characterized by thought disorder. Holzman, Shenton, and Solovay (1986) found that persons with mania and those with schizophrenia had distinctive types of thought disorder. In mania, they found loosely related ideas excessively combined and elabo-

42

rated; in schizophrenia, they found interpenetration of one idea by another, unstable referents, and the impression of inner turmoil. Andreasen and Grove (1986) also noted that those with affective illnesses differed in type of thought disorder from those with schizophrenia, as well as in the degree of improvement. They found that those with mania remitted best.

Thought disorder has at various times been attributed to a variety of factors—perceptual disorder, language disturbance, attentional deficit, and emotional disturbance (Cutting, 1985). Undoubtedly all of these factors are involved in some way, but there is no agreement as to which comes first or precisely how they may interact.

Clinicians and researchers have made many attempts to observe and describe thought disorder. Some have perceived it as an impaired association between ideas, resulting in impaired logic and confusion. Others have focused on issues relating to the use of abstractions. Some of these investigators have noted a limited capacity for abstract thinking and excessively concrete thought, whereas others have found thought processes to be excessively abstract (Johnston & Holzman, 1979).

Cameron (1944) proposed the term "overinclusiveness" for what he believed to be the fundamental disturbance in schizophrenic thinking. Overinclusiveness describes the inability to maintain conceptual boundaries, so that the irrelevant and tangential are included in the stream of thought. This leads to vagueness, confusion, and incomprehensibility. Others have noted an inability of patients to categorize appropriately and to focus on the most relevant aspects of a situation.

Only a few researchers (e.g., Freedman, 1974; Kaplan, 1964; Torrey, 1983) have focused on patients' own statements about their experiences in coping with cognitive difficulties. Patients in Freedman's study described themselves as "confused," "hazy," "bewildered," and "disoriented." They reported that they experienced blocking and sometimes felt their minds going blank, and that they were not able to maintain control over their own thought processes.

RACING THOUGHTS AND STIMULUS OVERLOAD

One of the dilemmas most frequently reported by people with schizophrenia is the experience of having thoughts racing through their heads in an uncontrollable fashion. They report feeling bombarded with stimuli and being unable to sort out the relevant from the irrelevant. This rush of idea leaves them confused and bewildered, and unable to carry out the tasks they have set for themselves (Freedman, 1974).

"What happened to me in Toronto," one patient related, "was a breakdown in the filter and a hodge-podge of unrelated stimuli were distracting me from things which should have had my undivided attention" (MacDonald, 1960, p. 218). Several patients have used the analogy of the loss of a "filtering system," which they feel normally protects people from this highly disturbing experience.

Carol North (1987) helps us understand the terrible reality of constant noise in a patient's head in her book *Welcome Silence*. After coping nearly all her life with the insistent intrusion of voices and other noises, North responded to a kidney dialysis treatment, and all the irrelevant noises disappeared. She concludes her book with a vivid contrast between the painful cacophony of sounds she endured for so many years and the "welcome silence" when her head became clear and she was able to direct her own thoughts.

Torrey (1983) believes the flooding of the mind with thoughts to be a consequence of overacuteness of the senses. It is as if the brain is being bombarded with both external and internal stimuli. Torrey quotes one patient as follows:

> My trouble is that I've got too many thoughts. You might think about something, let's say the ashtray, and just think, oh! yes, that's the thing for putting my cigarette in, but I would think of it and then I would think of a dozen other things connected with it at the same time. (p. 10)

Feeling flooded with thoughts leads some patients to believe that someone is inserting thoughts into their head. According to another of Torrey's informants,

> All sorts of "thoughts" seem to come to me, as if someone is "speaking" them inside my head. When in any company it appears to be worse (probably some form of self-consciousness). I don't want the "thoughts" to come but I keep on "hearing" them (as it were) and it requires a lot of will power sometimes to stop myself from "thinking" (in the form of "words") the most absurd and embarrassing things. (p. 11)

A patient choosing to remain anonymous wrote the following account of her experience with racing thoughts and her efforts in learning to manage them:

> Psychotic episodes have the effect of "playing" mental messages on 78 + and frequently switching stations. Disorganized thoughts are often best managed in organized environments. Impulsive obsessive–

compulsive behaviors have been a critical indicator that my mental
world is not well organized. I have learned to manage this by a
process I call "mental purging." (Anonymous, 1989b, p. 19)

Anonymous has learned to structure her life by making lists and setting priorities, and by giving herself reasonable time frames for getting things done. She has found writing to be a healthy form of coping,
for "it purges my mind of information that interferes with action and
helps to organize my thoughts into action patterns" (1989b, p. 19).
Eventually Anonymous returned to work and to graduate school, where
she had to struggle against great difficulties in learning to concentrate.
She persisted, and in time, especially after discontinuing medications,
became more proficient than she had been before her illness. She learned
through subsequent episodes that she could not push herself or allow
others to push her.

YIELDING TO ASSOCIATIVE CONNECTIONS

Some of the patients described by Freedman (1974) expressed great
difficulty staying on a topic, because each idea immediately and auto-
matically suggested a large number of associated ideas. They were unable to control this phenomenon and found that it seriously affected
their ability to concentrate. One patient provided the following example: "My thoughts wander around in circles without getting any-
where. I try to read even a paragraph in a book, but it takes me ages,
because each bit I read starts me thinking in ten different directions
at once" (Freedman, 1974, p. 335). Another of Freedman's subjects
reported that he was unable to read the newspaper because everything
he read had a large number of associations. Still another subject
described her inability to resist yielding to associations that made it
impossible for her to remember, read, or think: "I started a train of
ideas which finished itself or got lost in a tangle of cross-associa-
tions. . . . I could not direct its course at all" (1974, p. 335).
     From the outside, schizophrenic thought patterns appear discon-
nected, disorganized, and illogical. A view from the inside reveals how
they are experienced:

> My thoughts get all jumbled up, I start thinking about something
> but I never get there. Instead I wander off in the wrong direction
> and get caught up with all sorts of things that might be connected
> with the things I want to say but in a way I can't explain. People
> listening to me get more lost than I do. (Patient quoted in Torrey,
> 1983, p. 18)

Being plagued by loose and rapid associations and racing thoughts leaves some patients feeling frighteningly out of control. Their thoughts seem to take on an existence of their own, as in this patient's experience:

> My mind seemed almost to have a life and a direction of its own.
> . . . I became increasingly aware of the separate life of my own
> mind. Without informing me of its intentions, without thinking[,]
> which seemed to me the means by which . . . my mind allowed me
> to participate . . . I found myself doing things (except it was not
> thinking in the usual sense), there was no process of conscious
> deliberate thought. (Freedman, 1974, pp. 335–336)

Freedman (1974) felt that this sense of loss of voluntary control leads naturally to the delusional belief of being controlled by some external being, whose form and voice are then hallucinated.

The press of activity, loosening of inhibitory restraints, and distractibility are well-known characteristics of people suffering from mania. Landis and Mettler (1964) provided the following example of a patient's recollection of the experience of losing control and sliding into mania:

> One begins to slip; the world about one changes imperceptibly. For
> a time it is possible to keep some sort of grip on reality. But once
> one is really over the edge, once the grip of reality is lost, the forces
> of the Unconscious take charge, and then begins what appears to
> be an unending voyage into the universe of bliss or the universe of
> horror as the case may be. (p. 283)

SLOWED THOUGHTS AND MENTAL BLOCKING

Some people with mental illness report that they frequently experience mental exhaustion. They are simply too tired to continue thinking at all. This is an understandable consequence of trying to cope with racing thoughts and loose associations. Allied to mental exhaustion may be a marked retardation in thinking. Thoughts may follow one another at a snail's pace as the mind works slowly and painfully. One of Freedman's (1974) subjects likened the experience to a gramophone slowing down.

During depression, a patient's mind moves slowly and with much difficulty. Most of the time it is particularly impossible to think at all. All attempts to direct thoughts purposefully are diverted by the intrusion of hopelessness and helplessness. Dorothy Minor (1989) has told how when staff members were encouraged to carry on light conversation with patients, even such a simple question as "Do you live with your mother?" seemed too hard for her to answer. The experience of an individual quoted by Landis and Mettler (1964) further illustrates the point:

> Very often persons, places, and things, would occur to me, the names and particular appearances of which I was unable to recall without long endeavor of a most wearisome kind. I could not remember the name of some one, nor present to my fancy the faces or forms or various persons or things with which I had been familiar; nor could I banish them from my thoughts, but was constrained to use every method I could devise to bring to my remembrance what I was forced to pursue, until I alighted on the name or object that was suggested to me. Often when found, it would suggest to me something else of the same kind, with similar disquietude, till I felt that the labours of Sisyphus were less fatiguing and useless than those from which I could not escape. (p. 151)

Thought blocking is another commonly observed characteristic of schizophrenic thinking (Freedman, 1974; Torrey, 1983). It is experienced by patients as a sudden loss of all thoughts, as if the mind has just gone blank or had been emptied of everything. Patients may forget what they were about to say or may be left speechless in mid-sentence. Torrey (1983) quotes one such person as follows:

> For instance, I have often desired to open my mouth, and to address persons in different manners, and I have begun without premeditation a very rational and consecutive speech . . . but in the midst of my sentence, the power has either left me, or words have been suggested contradictory of those that went before; and I have been deserted, gaping, speechless, or stuttering in great confusion. (p. 22)

A number of Freedman's subjects reported a frightening "aphasic-like" diffuse loss of meaning of common words, objects, and people. This made their world seem unreal. In some cases, they could not remember who people were, or what their relationships with these people had meant to them. The loss of meaning sometimes extended to words, which then made no sense.

Martee Singleterry (personal communication, July 1, 1990) has explained how she suffers loss of meaning in a variety of situations. To begin with, as a child she realized she was different in some ways. While learning to read, she felt that she learned to say the words but was unable to put meaning to them. She had to teach herself to read later when she realized that she was not actually reading in any meaningful sense. Until she was in her 20s, English was not too meaningful to her; she pretty much had her own language until then. As an adult, Singleterry still has trouble associating names with faces. She sometimes has difficulty forming correct associations even with people with whom she should be quite familiar. She has learned to pick up cues from people as to their identity and to respond to expectations, so as to manage social situations adequately.

Torrey (1983) has identified a fundamental defect in the thinking of schizophrenic patients: They are unable to sort, synthesize, and respond in a normal fashion. They have difficulty synthesizing visual and auditory stimuli or in bringing the two together, as in these examples provided by Torrey's informants:

> I have to put things together in my head. If I look at my watch I see the watchstrap, watch, face, hands and so on, then I have got to put them together to get into one piece. (p. 15)

> I can't concentrate on television because I can't watch the screen and listen to what is being said at the same time. I can't seem to take in two things like this at the same time especially when one of them means watching and the other means listening. On the other hand I seem to be always taking in too much at the one time and then I can't handle it and can't make sense of it. (p. 15)

DISTURBANCES IN JUDGMENT AND REASONING

Although direct care providers and families would probably place illogical thinking and poor judgment high on the list of impairments in mental illness, Freedman (1974) found considerable disagreement among his informants on this subject. Some patients argued that their reasoning powers were unimpaired, but that they started from wrong premises. According to Landis and Mettler (1964), Clifford Beers argued in his book *The Mind That Found Itself* that contrary to what most "sane" people think, "insane" people do not necessarily think illogically; they may come to wrong conclusions by using perfect logic but incorrect premises. They use mental processes very much like those characteristic of well-ordered minds.

Others in Freedman's study felt that their reasoning was unimpaired, but that they reached false conclusions because their information came from disturbed perceptions. Some felt that their reasoning suffered from interference from hallucinations. Still others of Freedman's subjects did agree that their capacity to reason logically was impaired. One of his informants described it this way:

A parody of rational thought may be found, but true critical judgment is entirely lost. . . . My conscious mind is like an information center whose staff are sick; as more of them become incapacitated, so the rest become more severely overworked. To send them a mass of new material to be worked out at this moment makes disorganization complete. Reason clocks off and leaves the door open to the inner mind. Unconscious impulses, like a band of irresponsible children, take over the telephone exchange and play around with the controls. It may be weeks or even months before the responsible organizers are back at their places and order is restored. . . . I can sum up the process as follows: cerebral overstimulation, sectional failure of mental organization, chaos. (p. 337)

HOW PATIENTS COPE WITH
IMPAIRED COGNITIVE PROCESSES

Clearly, having one's thinking processes go so seriously awry has highly detrimental affects on all aspects of living. It appears from Chapter 3 that it can have a serious affect on a person's sense of self and his or her ability to exert control over these disturbances. To some extent this is true, but what is encouraging is how many people speak of making efforts to manage these symptoms and of developing strategies whereby they can go on with life.

Some of the patients quoted thus far in the chapter have told us how they exert great will power to stop themselves from thinking "the most absurd and embarrassing things"; how they manage obsessive thoughts by a process called "mental purging"; and how they structure life by making lists and setting reasonable time frames. One patient uses writing to "purge" her irrelevant thoughts and to organize her relevant thoughts into action patterns. Another identified her difficulty in putting meaning to the English language and taught herself to read and communicate meaningfully.

Probably the most frequently used coping strategy reported by this sample of subjects was that of creating structure for themselves. Many of them found it difficult to deal with their irrelevant thoughts directly, but they did find that quieter, calmer environments and knowing what to expect eased their anxieties and made it possible for them to function more optimally. For example, Esso Leete (1987a) has learned the following about her situation:

Stress plays a major role in my illness. Whatever I can do to decrease or avoid high stress situations or environments is helpful in controlling my symptoms. Too much free time, leisure time, I have found to be detrimental; regular structured activity, however is immeasurably important for my functioning and overall outlook in life, especially when combined with ongoing encouragement and support. When one has a chaotic inner existence, a predictable daily schedule is helpful. (p. 89)

Cathy King-Hasher (1989) remembered her highly beneficial experiences attending Catholic school when she was a child:

[I went to] Catholic school, starting in second grade. There I flourished in the steady, orderly environment. The rules were basic and few, and always enforced; the discipline was calm, firm, and consistent. . . . my talents bloomed and my achievements were considerable in the safety and freedom I experienced in this place. (p. 8)

Upon reaching adulthood, King-Hasher suffered a severe psychotic disorder. She recalled these successful early years in Catholic school and knew what she needed to do to function well:

I need order, structure, fairness and consistency in my environment and relationships, plenty of positive ways to use my mental and physical energy, strong values, and principles to order my thinking and action. Also I need clear communication and enough non-hostile, non-fussy attention from others . . . all of which (in my opinion) the rest of the world could use as well. (p. 9)

Martee Singleterry (personal communication, July 2, 1990) has found that her memory is not sufficiently dependable. She has devised a range of strategies to help her keep track of things and events, with the computer being the latest tool she has adapted to her use. A few years ago, Singleterry's insight into her handicap began bringing invitations by organizations and the mass media to speak publicly. Although she was interested in doing this, she was unable to organize her thoughts ahead of time in order to prepare a presentation. She made an adaptation to this problem, however, by requesting a change in format so that she would be asked specific questions, to which she was quite able to formulate responses. Singleterry sees her problem as a special kind of learning disability, and feels that professionals need to develop particular teaching strategies for helping people with problems like hers.

The theme throughout Carol North's (1987) autobiography is one of constant struggle to appear normal, to perform well in spite of the persistent intrusion of voices and bizarre thoughts. Since childhood she has spent an inordinate amount of time policing her thoughts to prevent them from escaping, and practicing "mental gymnastics" in order to make a normal external experience. She was an honor student in high school and eventually succeeded in getting her medical degree. This was possible only through grit, perseverance, and a variety of inventive coping strategies.

IMPLICATIONS FOR RESEARCH AND PRACTICE

We learn from patients that they experience cognitive confusion, bewilderment, and disorientation. They are often troubled with racing thoughts, loosened associations, attentional deficits, memory loss, and thought blocking. Many of these patients have actively analyzed their situation and created adaptive strategies to help them cope. They tend to see these difficulties as comcomitants of stress resulting from an excess of internal and external stimulation. Their coping strategies revolve around creating structure for themselves and avoiding environments that are toxic to them.

Professionals also see stress as a factor in schizophrenic thought disorder and poor functioning. Cutting (1985) notes that people with schizophrenia respond markedly to stress, tend to recover from automatic disturbances slowly, and are reactive to a broad range of anxiety-provoking stimuli. They also experience a failure of gating or filtering out of stimuli, which leads to distractibility and disorganization.

These observations have led to considerable attention to the question of which types of environments are most supportive of patient functioning. Although the focus has been first and foremost on the family, what has been learned can and should be transferred to all professionally provided services. A number of researchers have concluded that excessive stimulation in the home can lead to patient relapse and that family therapy aimed at reducing stress may result in better outcome (Anderson et al., 1986; Falloon, Boyd, & McGill, 1984; Leff & Vaughn, 1985; Strachan, 1986). Questions about this research continue to arise (Hatfield, Spaniol, & Zipple, 1987; Lefley, 1992; Kanter, Lamb, & Loeper, 1987), but the evidence for patients' vulnerability to stress is rarely questioned.

Although the stress of greatest concern in the above-described research is that resulting from "critical comments" and "overinvolvement," patient statements and observations by others have identified a variety of potential stressors for this population. Pepper and Ryglewicz (1986), for example, believe that people with schizophrenia lack an adequate stimulus barrier and are thus vulnerable to many kinds of stimuli. They see many of the behaviors of mentally ill people as efforts to adapt to these impairments, with some approaches, such as excessive withdrawal, acting-out behavior, and alcohol and drug abuse, leading to dysfunction.

Pepper and Ryglewicz note further that stimulation cannot be measured on a single axis. Any attempt to assess the amount of stimulation must consider kind and quality of stimulation as well as quantity, and it must attend to the meaning an event has for a person. Even though the stimulation from the outside may be mild, there may be considerable reaction because of the way it relates to what is going on inside the person. The fantasy or delusional system can be an amplifier and/or a distorter of experience.

The number of stimuli impinging on an individual at a given time can also play a part in determining the level of stress experienced, as people with schizophrenia have great difficulty selecting out what they should be attending to. Yet another factor is the degree of familiarity of the stimuli to the individual. Unfamiliar stimuli can be a threat to the person's sense of competence and self-esteem.

Pepper and Ryglewicz (1986) postulate that each individual has a minimum acceptable level and a maximum tolerable level of activity and sensory stimulation. There may be a wide range between the two for healthy people, but for people with mental illnesses the range may be very constricted, leaving them easily incapacitated when the acceptable levels are exceeded. These authors' amplification of the meaning of stress and stress tolerance has considerable applicability to the provision of environments for mentally ill men and women everywhere. Hospitals, clinics, residential and psychosocial services, and family homes all need to consider how they can best structure their environments to permit maximum cognitive functioning.

From the psychosocial field, we learn that the field of psychiatric rehabilitation now has its own conceptual base, which is the "vulnerability–stress–coping–competence model" (Anthony & Liberman, 1986; Liberman, 1986; Liberman et al., 1986). In general, the aims of an approach based on this model are (1) to teach mentally ill individuals specific skills to aid them in coping with their environments, and (2) to develop environmental resources to support and strengthen the individuals' functioning. Effective coping with life's stressors involves particular skills to enable the mentally ill person to master the challenges and problems inherent in daily living. In addition, most family education and consultation programs give considerable training to families in creating benign, supportive environments for their mentally ill relatives (Bernheim & Lehman, 1985; Hatfield, 1990). Hatfield (1990, p. 119) characterizes a supportive environment as one that provides the following:

- Continuity and predictability
- Adequate structure and form
- Limited amount and intensity of stimulation
- Clear and calm communications
- Appropriate expectations
- Encouragement and positive regard

It should be noted that up to this point the emphasis in our discussion has been on indirect approaches to helping people with cognitive dysfunction. A possible third and more direct way of helping people with thinking disorders is to identify the nature of the impairment and to attempt to treat it directly.

Cutting (1985) reports that the revival of cognitive psychology has resulted in a growth of information-processing and cognitive theories of schizophrenia. Several studies have attempted to modify delusions and hallucinations by cognitive methods. Although these methods were more commonly used before the introduction of neuroleptics, they have been reconsidered for patients who do not respond to medications. Watts, Powell, and Austin (1975) developed a method for belief modification based on the following principles: Begin with the most weakly held belief, avoid direct confrontation, discuss the evidence for the belief rather than the belief itself, and encourage the person to bring up counterarguments.

Cognitive therapy for depressed patients has been well established, with the best-articulated and researched being that of Beck and associates (Beck, Rush, Shaw, & Emery, 1979). In general, their therapy focuses on negative thinking patterns that cause people to become depressed or maintain their depressions once they have started. Beck et al. have identified a number of types of cognitive distortions, such as overgeneralization, magnification, minimization, and arbitrary inference. These and other cognitive distortions seem to be associated with schizophrenia as well, but treatment development in this area is still minimal.

Goldberg and Cook (1990), drawing from the field of neuropsychology, believe that attention needs to be given to the reasons for loss of functioning in schizophrenia. They question the efficacy of psychosocial techniques that focus exclusively on behavior, with no concern for the underlying processes that produce the handicap. They note that many common features of schizophrenia significantly interfere with the learning process: the positive symptoms of delusions and hallucinations, the limited capacity of the brain to hold information, the disorders of attention and memory, and the inability to plan. They are exploring the possibilities for cognitive remediation of some of these deficits by focusing on the processes rather than the content of schizophrenic thinking.

Perhaps, as Weiss (1989) has noted in a recent paper, conceptualizations that rely almost solely on symptoms are inadequate to a cognitive approach to schizophrenia. The enormous research literature in the field has been of little usefulness to practitioners. The author believes that we need to build bridges between observable symptoms and the underlying processes (e.g., information processing, attention, and arousal) that produce them, and that we now have the scientific methodology to study these processes. The study of underlying processes has the advantage of tending to be measurable in the absence of the psychosis. Most (if not all) schizophrenic patients do not have normal cognitive functioning, even when in remission. The subliminal processes that tend to underlie the psychosis may be the more fruitful subjects for investigation (Weiss, 1989).

SUMMARY

In summary, we have found that patients' perceptions of the kinds of factors most conducive to better cognitive functioning can lead us to useful guidelines for creating supportive environments. All service agencies need to keep in mind the necessity for low stimulation, adequate structure, and clear unambiguous communication. Although it is less common for patients to identify specific cognitive impairments, some clinicians are beginning to focus on these underlying processes, with the expectation that a more direct cognitive remediation is ultimately possible.

CHAPTER FIVE

Disturbances in Emotions, Relationships, and Behaviors

Disturbances in emotions run the gamut in serious mental illnesses. Patients report experiencing exaggerated feelings of fear, anxiety, depression, guilt, and a variety of physical pains; sometimes they experience the opposite, with little or no feeling at all. These disturbances in emotions—together with abberrations in perceptual and cognitive functioning, not to mention a confused sense of self—inevitably result in impaired interpersonal relationships and inappropriate behaviors.

DISTURBANCES IN EMOTIONS

Although Torrey (1983) does not believe that exaggerated feelings are usually found in schizophrenia beyond the early stages, and although DSM-III-R (American Psychiatric Association, 1987) does not identify exaggerated emotions as a primary characteristic of schizophrenia, patients diagnosed with schizophrenia—as well as those with mood disorders and severe anxiety disorders—do report suffering highly disabling emotional experiences. For example, Anonymous (1989c), in a short article entitled "Problems of Living with Schizophrenia," has stated:

> The largest problem I face—I think the basic one—is the intensity and variety of my feelings, and my low threshold for handling other people's intense feelings, especially negative ones. I have often experienced a euphoric "high" that is much like being in contact with some greater reality or meaning to life—accompanied by a kind of added brightness or extra dimension to everyday things around me. The other side of the coin, though, is a very intense anxiety from nowhere that typically hits me quite suddenly after a short period of time without medication. The two feelings are opposite, yet somehow connected. (p. 4)

Fear and Anxiety

According to some authorities, fear and anxiety usually accompany depression and schizophrenia, and may be among the most disabling components of these disorders (Cutting, 1985; Landis & Mettler, 1964). Fear and anxiety, of course, are the primary symptoms in anxiety disorders. Terror, apprehension, horror, and depersonalization are frequent. Fear may be blended with other emotional states, such as unreality, anger, or reverence. There may be feelings of impending death, disease, or disaster. Fears can be all-pervasive and all-powerful, blotting out all other feelings and interests. When in the throes of fear the whole person is immobilized, even while seeking a center of safety. Torrey (1983) has noted that when people with schizophrenia suffer from extreme fears and anxieties, these tend to be pervasive, nameless, and without object. This seems to have been the case in the following accounts:

> Suddenly Fear, agonizing, boundless fear, overcame me, not the usual uneasiness of unreality, of calamity. . . . Outwardly, however, no one suspected the inquietude or the fear. People thought I was hysterical or manic. (Sechehaye, 1951, pp. 13–14)

> My fear was based fundamentally upon a terror of myself, of what was happening to me, of the helplessness that was overpowering my faculties. . . . I began to be afraid of people, of my family and friends; not because of what they represented, I soon learned, but because of my own inability to cope with ordinary human contacts. (Patient quoted in Landis & Mettler, 1964, p. 251)

Landis and Mettler (1964) selected the following patient's account to illustrate a case of "melancholia" accompanied by fear:

> There is no emotion in life more paralyzing than fear, no element more devastating. It is the archenemy of man and from the time [my illness started] until I recovered it was my constant companion. I learned to know it in all its aspects, real and imaginary, and as it stalked my footsteps I did not have to look back to be aware of its presence for its heavy chill hand was always on my shoulder. (p. 250)

Whether anxiety in mental illness is a primary symptom that gives rise to psychotic thought or whether anxiety is a consequence of the psychotic experience has been debated (Cutting, 1985). In one experience, that of Anonymous (1955), it seemed to be a consequence of it. Anonymous believed that he or she had discovered the secrets of the universe and was embarked on a great Promethean adventure. The person felt audacious and unconquerable until his or her first hospitalization:

> Shortly after I was taken to the hospital for the first time in a rigid catatonic condition, I was plunged into the horror of a world of cataclysm and totally dislocated. I myself have been responsible for setting the destructive forces into motion, although I had acted with no intent to harm and defended myself with healthy indignation against the accusations of others. (p. 680)

People with schizophrenia use huge amounts of energy trying to manage their anxieties. Thus they are tired and worn out all the time, and have great difficulty coping with the ordinary tasks of daily living. Mendel (1974) has recommended that professionals learn to teach anxiety management techniques. He has found that when a patient has developed techniques for anxiety management, other symptoms recede. Such techniques can be taught, he believes, by example, cognitive learning, and specific instruction.

Depression

Depression is the central difficulty in mood disorders, but depressed mood is also common in schizophrenia. Some authorities feel that there is a "shared pathophysiological mechanism," with depression being an integral part of schizophrenia as well as mood disorders. Others feel that depression in schizophrenia is a reaction to the psychotic state when insight returns. Still others feel that some depressions are reactive to medications (see Cutting, 1985).

The person who is severely depressed feels sad, despondent, and overcome with despair and hopelessness. There may be disturbances in sleeping and eating, as well as a markedly diminished interest in things once found pleasurable. The depressed person also often experiences loss of energy, diminished ability to concentrate, and recurrent thoughts of death (American Psychiatric Association, 1987).

Although there are many commonalities in the accounts of depression we have included here, there are also many individual and unique aspects that require our attention. In the account written by Norma MacDonald, one of Kaplan's (1964) informants, actual physical pain accompanied her depression:

> I reached a stage where almost my entire world consisted of tortured contemplation of things which brought pain and uncontrol-

lable depression. My brain after a short time, became sore with a real physical soreness, as if it had been rubbed with sand paper until it was raw. It felt like a bleeding sponge. (Kaplan, 1964, p. 176)

Another patient who provided an account for Kaplan, John Custance, said that a profound revulsion accompanied his depressions:

> When in a depressive period I have an intense revulsion to lavatories, excreta, urine, or anything associated with them. This revulsion extends to all kinds of dirt. I loathe going to the lavatory, using a chamber pot, or touching anything the least bit dirty. (Kaplan, 1964, p. 48)

George Fish (1985), mental health advocate and free-lance writer, has described his depression less in terms of sadness and more in terms of despair and nothingness:

> Being chronically depressed is like being trapped inside a bare, white room, a seamless monotony from which there is no escape. In fact, it is this which is the essence of depression: the despair of absolute *nothingness*, of being trapped in a complete void. Nothingness: that is depression—no color, no light, no spirit, no substance, no reality, no fantasy, just the paralyzing sense of despair that nothing, *absolutely nothing* can be done to change it. (p. 2; emphasis the author's)

Another person who has experienced profound nothingness and despair, Nancy Young Chevalier, published an extensive description of her experience in the "Health" section of the *Washington Post* (January 16, 1990):

> My broken brain causes me to feel abnormally, often interminably, depressed. I simply have no feelings—good, bad or indifferent. A nuclear bomb could be dropped on downtown Washington near my home; my family could be killed in a plane accident; I could win the Pulitzer Prize—it would all be the same to me. I, who normally read the daily paper at least for an hour, no longer know or care about what is happening in the world, or indeed in my own home. I do not bathe or dress; I move only from bedroom to the bathroom, or sometimes appear in the kitchen when no one is home and spread some peanut butter on a slice of bread. I know something to be dreadfully wrong but feel completely passive and helpless to do anything about it. (pp. 12–14)

Chevalier found help through a local support group, where she learned that doctors, pills, and therapies were not enough. She would have to build up her own response to this devastating illness. In addition to taking medication, she began to do yoga, walk every day, do volunteer work, and write creatively. She began listening to all kinds of music, and, when all else failed, imagined herself waltzing in Vienna.

Profound despair and the critical need for hope are evident in a poignant poem entitled "God Bless the Ground," written by Evonne Newman (1989):

> Here I stand, like a knight in my suit of heavy armour.
> It's a burden I didn't choose, but one I must bear.
>
> When I walk the suit is cumbersome.
> Therefore my steps are slow,
> That's the reason I walk on level ground.
>
> There's times I can't lift my head up,
> to see a blue sky above,
> so I look at the ground below.
>
> Yes, I look at the ground below with ease and see a lone flower
> insignificant to some,
> Yet, gloriously "hope" awakens within me again . . .
>
> "Hope," such a small word,
> yet its meaning is as a mighty sword
> to be used in this battle called "depression." (p. 3)

Landis and Mettler (1964) provided the following example of an individual with agonizing experiences of sleeplessness and fatigue:

> I was seized with an unspeakable physical weariness. There was a tired feeling in my muscles unlike anything I had ever experienced. A peculiar sensation appeared to travel up my spine to my brain. I had an indescribable nervous feeling. . . . I lay with dry, staring eyes gazing into space. I had a fear that some terrible calamity was about to happen. I grew afraid to be alone. (p. 262)

Guilt

Feelings of worthlessness and of excessive and inappropriate guilt are often found in depressed patients. It is as though they have committed an unpardonable sin for which no atonement is possible:

> Moral tensions returned in full force. I am haunted by a sense of guilt; my conscience gives me no rest, even when there do not seem to be any particularly grievous sins upon it. Whatever I am doing I feel I ought to be doing something else. I worry perpetually about

my past sins and failure; not for a moment can I forget the mess
I seem to have made of my life. However I may pray for forgive-
ness, no forgiveness comes. Eventually the terrors of Hell approach.
(Patient quoted in Landis & Mettler, 1964, pp. 4–5)

The pain and anguish of living with unrelieved guilt without cause or
explanation are further elucidated by one of Torrey's (1983) informants:

Later, considering them appropriate, I no longer felt guilty about
these fantasies, nor did the guilt have an actual object. It was too
pervasive, too enormous, to be founded on anything definite, and
it demanded punishment. The punishment was indeed horrible,
sadistic—it consisted fittingly enough of being guilty. For to feel
oneself guilty is the worst thing that can happen, it is the punishment of punishments. Consequently, I could never be relieved of
it as though I had been truly punished. Quite the reverse, I felt more
and more guilty. Constantly, I sought to discover what was punishing me so dreadfully, what was making me so guilty. (p. 36)

Mania

The essential feature of a manic episode is a distinct period when the
predominant mood is either elevated, expansive, or irritable. Associated
symptoms include inflated self-esteem, grandiosity, decreased need for
sleep, pressure of speech, flight of ideas, distractibility, and psycho-
motor agitation. Manic speech is typically loud, rapid, and difficult
to interpret.

I talked, laughed, cried, sang, shouted and danced to my heart's
content. The giving up of all attempt at self-control brought the
needed rest and sleep. The condition of my mind for many months
is beyond all description. My thoughts ran with lightning-like rapid-
ity from one subject to another. I had an exaggerated feeling of self-
importance. All the problems of the universe came crowding into
my mind, demanding instant discussion and solution—mental
telepathy, hypnotism, wireless telegraphy. (Patient quoted in Landis
& Mettler, 1964, p. 49)

Apathy, Blunting, and Inappropriate Affect

The most typical schizophrenic phenomena, according to some authorities, are blunting or flattening of affect, inappropriate affect, anhedo-
nia, and apathy (Cutting, 1985; Torrey, 1983). Sometimes, as in the

following case, it seems as though there is an exhaustion of feeling after having suffered too much and too long:

> Nothing interests me any longer. I am weary of everything—to be interested in nothing is unsupportable; it makes me nervous. Nothing is worth the trouble of the effort. I can no longer even get angry, for nothing is worth getting angry about, and I am astonished when I see people who have the courage to get angry. (Patient quoted in Landis & Mettler, 1964, p. 326)

Bleuler (1911/1950) gave considerable attention to what he perceived as inappropriate affect—incongruity among facial expression, speech, and activity. This also included such things as laughing upon hearing unpleasant news. The judgment of inappropriateness, however, comes from the observer. The patient's responses may be quite appropriate to the inner reality he or she is experiencing:

> Half the time I am talking about one thing and thinking about half a dozen other things at the same time. It must look queer to people when I laugh about something that has got nothing to do with what I am talking about, but they don't know what's going on inside and how much of it is running round in my head. You see I might be talking about something quite serious to you and other things come into my head at the same time that are funny and this makes me laugh. If I could only concentrate on the one thing at the one time I wouldn't look so silly. (Patient quoted in Torrey, 1983, p. 37)

Some patients describe a state of "just feeling," to which they cannot assign a specific emotion (e.g., anger, love, or fear). This usually occurs during an acute phase of the illness.

> Lying there I came as close, I think, as I ever have to a state of emotion unaccompanied by thoughts. I simply felt. Again, I have never learned words to describe sensations so far removed from what is called normal. General misery, physical discomfort, degradation not born of intellectual concept, but a deep, bodily and inner mental state; a feeling of being lost, lost utterly with no sense of place or time, no idea as to whom voices belonged, lost to light and form and color; a distinct, acid nausea of self-revulsion—all these were in the feeling that swept over me. (Patient quoted in Landis & Mettler, 1964, p. 321)

Bouricius (1989), a mother of a 32-year-old schizophrenic son ill for 12 years, has recently presented an interesting challenge to the view that people with schizophrenia are devoid of emotional responsiveness. Five mental health professionals who had known the son well over a period of many years rated the son on Andreasen's Scale for the Assessment of Negative Symptoms. There was general agreement among the raters that the young man did indeed score moderately high on a range of characteristics indicating affective flattening, inappropriate affect, poverty of speech, lack of ability to feel intimacy, and other characteristics usually classified as negative symptoms.

These ratings were compared to the personal statements the patient made in a collection of writings over a number of years, in which a significantly different picture emerged. In them were revealed a young man's intensely felt pain and loneliness as he cycled through years of psychotic illness. Certainly there is no lack of feeling in such statements as "Pain is in my chest. Sorrow is in my head and neck. Anguish is in my shoulders. All suffering is truly in me" (quoted in Bouricius, 1989, p. 204) or "Loneliness needs a song, a song of love and pain, sweet release and hope for the future. . . . Loneliness needs a song to fill the emptiness with tears and sighs and soothe the agony" (p. 207).

As the mother studied these writings, she found that at times her son seemed to be trying to shield himself from the intensity of his emotions in order to avoid becoming acutely psychotic. At other times he actually seemed to seek a psychotic state to avoid slipping into a state of absence of feeling. Bouricius has raised the question of whether many patients seen as lacking in affect may not really be experiencing strong emotions. She cautions that the Scale for the Assessment of Negative Symptoms may actually contribute to mental health professionals' failure to understand what is really going on within a person.

DISTURBANCES IN RELATIONSHIPS AND BEHAVIORS

People with schizophrenia are seen as unsociable, eccentric, suspicious, and solitary—often from childhood. They have poor empathy with other people, are rigid in behavior, communicate in unusual styles, and prefer to be alone. Some authorities think that this shut-in personality style, with its oversensitivity, reclusiveness, and reticence, may be attributable to constitutional factors (Cutting, 1985).

Mendel (1974) has talked of the "disastrously painful interpersonal transaction" (p. 40) of people with schizophrenia, and has ascribed them to their lack of historicity and difficulties in anxiety management. Their problems are aggravated by difficulties in establishing ego boundaries and by their chronically impaired self-esteem.

DeVries and Delespaul (1989) stress the need for systematic studies of schizophrenic patients' responses to social contexts, because they are known to be "environmentally vulnerable" and they tend to respond maladaptively to stressful social situations. Studies are needed in order to understand these patients' illnesses, plan treatments, and create optimal living environments. DeVries and Delespaul used the Experience Sampling Method to study nine patients in depth, and found that people with schizophrenia spent more time alone and that crowded situations were extremely troublesome for them. However, they did not respond well to being alone for long periods of time and reported feeling lonely and depressed. They felt best in small groups of two or three.

Patients' statements about interpersonal relations are somewhat less abundant in the available material than are statements about cognition and emotions. This seems to confirm observations of isolation and lack of interest in other people, but this is by no means universally true; some of these writings contain some very poignant and revealing statements.

The complexity of the problem of intimacy in schizophrenia has been revealed by the following anonymous patient:

> Intimacy is an interesting problem in my life. In a way, I am capable of the deepest spiritual intimacy with people, yet, I am less capable than most people of handling the demands of relationships. I cannot share negative feelings other people have, because I am too sensitive to them: yet I can give a great deal of love and concern when I am protected against feelings like anger and cynicism. (Anonymous, 1989c, p. 5)

Acute awareness of other people's feelings complicates life for those who are environmentally sensitive. The same anonymous individual notes that other people's feelings are more problematic when they are partly concealed or ambiguous and when the person is required to assume a socially accepted facade.

> Problems with my normal "facade" arise mainly when other people expect me to become emotionally involved with them. I find emotions tremendously complex, and I am quite acutely aware of the many over- and undertones of things people say and the way they say them. Generally, I like direct, honest, kind people, and I have difficulty handling social situations that require me to be artificial or too careful. (Anonymous, 1988c, p. 5)

Marcia Lovejoy (1989), who became an early and outspoken advocate for the mentally ill following many years in various institutions, found that other patients were a source of great support to her. Lovejoy puzzled about staff members' discouraging friendships among patients because they thought the patients reinforced one another's illnesses, when it was her experience that they gave one another support and help. She has said, "I could not confide my problems with hallucinations, or my fears about the FBI, to anyone who had not had similar experiences" (p. 25). She felt that other patients understood her sense of shame, anger, and fear.

Capacity for friendship was reported by yet another anonymous patient in a highly amusing and light-hearted fashion, rare in the first-person accounts that we have reviewed. The author describes in considerable detail her first meeting with "Penny," their various antics in the mental hospital, and their long association after discharge. She said, "Penny brought laughter and happiness. She was generous—willing me an oil well—in hopes of lifting the darkness and relieving the pain. She came into my life like a personal Santa Claus" (Anonymous, 1989, p. 2). This story surely suggests that not every person diagnosed with schizophrenia suffers from an inability to relate. What we do not know, of course, are the reasons for the great differences among patients in this behavior.

Probably no one in our collection of patient statements has stated the agony of loneliness more poignantly than the schizophrenic son of Bouricius (1989). Quotation after quotation indicates the search for love and relatedness that inevitably eluded this patient:

> I am a lonely nothing, a being, but pass me by. Forever pass me by. Strangers, I don't see you. My afflictions fill the place that was meant for sharing love. I am crying in despair. (p. 202)

> I cannot control what words do to me. My physiology weeps. I hate myself. I am too weak to apologize for hurting the world. I want to love. I envy those who can relate to each other. I have a dreadful fear of not loving, of not living, of not dying. (p. 205)

It is quite probable that most people in the depths of acute psychosis are so fully immersed in their internal activity that they have little inclination or ability to concern themselves about other people. Sommer and Osmond (1960) noted little tendency for patients to compare their psychotic experiences. Presumably each experience is considered so unique, so ineffable, that it could not be comprehended by others. This has led the authors to question the benefits of group therapy.

However, it may well be that this apparent lack of interest in others occurs primarily during times of greater preoccupation with florid symptoms, and that the desire for human contact is there at other times.

One might conclude this to be true from a recent study done by Leggatt (1986) of members of the Schizophrenia Fellowship of Australia. Leggatt surveyed patients' perceptions of their most difficult symptoms of the past and what they were now experiencing. Patients said that the most troublesome symptoms of the past were disorders of feeling and thinking. With 95% of the patients now on neuroleptics, these symptoms were reported less often; more concern was expressed in the present about the loss of concentration, loss of motivation, loss of confidence, and a sense of loneliness (Leggatt, 1986).

Leggatt reported that the problem of interpersonal relationships for many patients was compounded by their discomfort at having to associate with "mad people." They objected to the less disturbed being mixed in with the severely disturbed and young people with the elderly, and they complained about the lack of privacy when their mental states were most precarious. Hatfield (1989), using family members as informants, found the same desire for more homogeneous groupings of clients in psychosocial programs. Families felt that their relatives' unwillingness to enter a program or dropping out later could often be attributed to an unacceptable mix of people in age and functionality.

Some of the interpersonal disturbances in schizophrenia may also be present in other psychiatric diagnoses such as bipolar and depressive disorders. People with these disorders also tend to be environmentally sensitive, hypersensitive to the behaviors of others, and uncomfortable in social situations.

Clarkin and Haas (1988) have summarized some of the interpersonal difficulties of people with DSM-III-R affective disorders. They note that many individuals with these disorders tend to be insecure in social situations and constantly seek recognition and approval. They are easily hurt by disapproval and may react to criticism with rage, shame, and humiliation. Argumentativeness, inappropriate sexually seductive behavior, and self-centeredness get in the way of satisfying interpersonal relationships with others.

Family members often report a wide range of difficult patient behaviors as great sources of burden and stress for them. They identify such problems as argumentativeness; excesses in smoking, eating, and sleeping; self-destructive behaviors; running away; isolation; medication noncompliance; and a host of other problems as sources of special difficulty (Hatfield, 1990; Hatfield & Lefley, 1987). Although patients occasionally mention these behaviors, indicating that they are aware of them, they rarely seem to be aware of their effects on others. Explanations probably lie in their profound involvement in their own inner turmoil, their inability to take the roles of others, and a feeling of being victims of environmental forces rather than players in creating them.

IMPLICATIONS FOR RESEARCH AND PRACTICE

Accounts of patients with schizophrenia raise many questions about how reliably we interpret what they are experiencing. While traditionally we have thought these patients to be low in affect and lacking in interest in relating to others, our patient accounts suggest that there are many exceptions to this generally held belief. Questions also arise in regard to what is thought to be inappropriate affect. Laughing out loud, for example, may be perfectly appropriate in the context of the inner world, but appear bizarre in the social context of the moment.

Interpersonal relationships are seriously disturbed in depressive illnesses as well as in schizophrenia. In a depressive state, feelings of worthlessness, hopelessness, and guilt can be so overwhelming that the individual is incapable of interacting with others. Families and friends feel helpless in penetrating the gloom that encompasses the depressed person.

Treatments emphasizing psychosocial rehabilitation are being developed to address issues of interpersonal relationships and behaviors of people with mental illnesses (Liberman, 1986; Anthony & Liberman, 1986). Although these approaches are probably now most often based on behaviors that are exhibited by clients, we believe that their effectiveness can be considerably enhanced by increased understanding of the inner experiences of these individuals.

While people with schizophrenia and affective disorders claim to be exquisitively sensitive to their interpersonal environments, families and friends often feel misunderstood and neglected. This suggests that some people with mental illnesses may have difficulty interpreting the feelings of others or may magnify the intensity of feelings being expressed by others. Perhaps these are areas in which psychosocial treatments can offer remediation.

Finally, anxiety seems to be such a central problem for those with any of the major illnesses that we need to give it our attention. It would be helpful if we knew whether anxiety is a core deficit that results in or aggravates other symptoms of these illnesses, or whether anxiety is a reaction to the many dilemmas of living with these disorders. This may lead us to teach anxiety management more effectively, as Mendel (1974) has advocated.

CHAPTER SIX

Cruising the Cosmos, Part Three: Psychosis and Hospitalization
A Consumer's Personal Recollection

FREDERICK J. FRESE, III, Ph.D.

What an exciting day this is. As I write, it is Sunday and it is Earth Day, April 22, 1990. It is the first beautiful spring day in the final decade of the second millennium. We are in the beginning days of the ebb of the Anglo-American cultural–linguistic economic empire, and I am in my home in Ohio, the Buckeye State, "the heart of it all." And I have an exciting challenge before me. I am being given an opportunity to describe something about the thought processes and experiences of a schizophrenic person, in writing to an audience consisting, I presume, primarily of "chronically normal persons" (CNPs). In that I have often stated that having a schizophrenic break is in some way like visiting an alien world where the customs and language structure are very different, I find this attempt to describe that world a real challenge.

Let me explain about the title of this chapter. I refer to "the cosmos" because I find that other consumers, in describing their experiences, often use this term. When I was returning from the National Consumers' Conference in Huntington, West Virginia, a few years ago, another psychologist/consumer and I were trying to explain to the two CNP social workers who were riding us about how our thought processes were different from theirs. After several inadequate attempts, I finally said that the major difference between us and them was that when they get overwhelmed, they may become tired, frustrated, or angry. We do that as well, of course, but we also have another option available: We can "alter the cosmos." The CNPs did not seem to understand very well, but I felt my metaphor had a strong ring of truth to it.

Two weeks ago, I was in Youngstown, Ohio, to hear a talk by Carol North. Dr. North (1987), now a board-certified psychiatrist, does an excellent job of describing her perceptions during the years she was schizophrenic. She says that while she was receiving the hemodialysis treatments that cured her, she was quite confident that any such physical treatments would be useless because she knew her problem was that she was at the "cosmic junction," and she was convinced that all she needed was to be moved away from it. At the time she was quite positive that medical interventions were unnecessary, and indeed totally irrelevant, when one is in what she calls "the parallel reality."

Likewise, I see that the consumer David Zelt (1989), in his fascinating *Schizophrenia Bulletin* article (now a book chapter), tells us that during his schizophrenic break colors took on special meanings. Green meant that he was like Christ, white represented spiritual purity, and the color orange indicated that he was attuned to "the cosmos."

With such precedents, I feel comfortable in sticking to the "cosmos" metaphor during this tale of recollection of my adventures in the world of schizophrenia.

I am employing the term "Part Three" in the title because this chapter focuses on my third major breakdown. I have already described my first two breakdowns in some detail in presentations at the National Consumers' Conference in Columbia, South Carolina, and at the annual meeting of the American Psychological Association in New Orleans. Both these meetings were held in the summer of 1989. A brief description of my first breakdown was published in the *APA Monitor* (Buie, 1989), and a University of Kansas psychology professor is now publishing expanded descriptions of my first two breakdowns in his forthcoming text on abnormal psychology (Holmes, 1991). Briefly, in my first episode I came to believe that Chinese Communists had hypnotized many Marines who had been fighting against them in Korea, and that the Chinese were about to take control of our military establishment by activating the hypnotized Marines who were under their power. The delusion was really not very creative, being very similar to the tale woven in the Frank Sinatra film *The Manchurian Candidate*, which I had seen a few years previously.

In my second breakdown, a year or two later, I had been able to secure employment working as a management trainee for a large Fortune 500 conglomerate. A few months after beginning work, I started to "understand" that all decisions could be made by translating the decision-making process into numerical codes. I decoded many of the problems that I knew the corporation was having, but unfortunately in the process, I myself started turning into various animals, in an evolutionary descending manner. I spent brief periods of time as an ape, a dog, a dragon or snake, a fish, an insect, and an amoeba; finally, I was turned into an atom in the inside of a nuclear explosive device that was on its way to destroy the Soviet Union and the rest of the world as well. Because Dr. Holmes is being kind enough to publish more details on these first two adventures, I use my space in this chapter to concentrate on "Adventure Number Three."

I am finding the writing of this document most exciting, not because I have the opportunity to describe for you my recollection of the third breakdown, but also because I am currently in a state that is beginning the process of going into schizophrenic thought. Because I have my pills and am quite confident that I can stop the process before it goes too much farther, this condition does not frighten me. But I think you may find that my surplus use of metaphors, rhymes, alliterations, and other modes of paleological logic may impress you as somewhat on the border of being "bizarre." You see, I have just returned from a 3-hour "gig" in Columbus, where I gave a "spill-the-guts" presentation to members of the Ohio Psychological Association. I frequently become more "schizophrenic" when faced with the excitement of a conference anyway, but I am finding that as I make self-revealing presentations, the excitement particularly intensifies. Right now, however, that may be an advantage because you, the reader, may be able to observe how a schizophrenic mind functions—not only from what I am writing about, but also from the way in which I describe things.

Enough of the preliminaries. Let me now take you with me into the cosmos. I am well seated in my silicone-chip electronic chariot, and my fingers are ready to fly over the keys as we visit the world of a metaphorical maelstrom. I will try to keep us in balance as we dart about. You may want to think of it as something like zooming about in a strange place, much as they do in George Lucas's *Star Wars* films.

We will go back to the summer of 1968. It was the weekend of the Fourth of July, and I was living in a large house at 143 Frambes Avenue, about two blocks east of the north side of the Ohio State University campus. There were 15 of us living in the house. The other 14 men in the house were veterans, graduate students, or both. Three doctoral students in astronomy lived on the top floor. The rest of us were crowded into rooms on the first and second floor. On the first floor there were a kitchen and two common areas, one of them the living room.

It had been about 6 months since I had returned to Columbus

after my second breakdown. During that time I had taken many job interviews with major corporations. I had a graduate degree in international management, and could speak passable Spanish and Japanese. I had taken numerous job interviews in both Columbus and New York. I had met some nice people in the process, but I also discovered that many, if not all, of the firms I interviewed with had policies against hiring persons recently released from mental hospitals. I had managed to obtain a job after about 3 months selling real estate for a firm in the northern part of town, but the only pay was commissions, and in the first 3 months I had not been able to sell or list any houses that sold. I was beginning to fear that I might never be able to work productively again.

As I remember it, the fellows in the house were having a big Fourth of July party. In readying myself for the party, for some reason I got it in my mind that I should dress my very best. Something was telling me that this was going to be a very special day. I went to my room and put on one of the two tailor-made suits that I had purchased when I was working for the Fortune 500 firm. I also put on my almost-new Florsheim Imperial wing-tipped shoes and the best tie I owned. This was very unusual for me, in that I ordinarily did not pay too much attention to my attire, and particularly since our Fourth of July party was to be a picnic and everyone else was to be dressed in a casual manner. But something told me this day was to be special. I remember going into the back yard and beginning to mingle with the other occupants of the house and our guests. During one conversation someone asked me what I did for a living. This was beginning to be a very difficult question for me to handle, because I was not earning any money. But I did have a real estate license and was attached to a realty company.

I remember that I responded to the question about my employment by saying, "I put people in homes." For some reason I started thinking that this was the funniest answer I had ever heard in my life. I started laughing. And I kept laughing. Everyone else was laughing with me. "I put people in homes." I did not know why it was so funny. Maybe it was because I had been "put in homes" for mental patients. I know that the laughing was great. It made me feel good for the first time since my breakdown 9 months before.

Now I was feeling very good. I was dressed in my best, I was making people laugh, and I knew it was going to be very special day. It was going to be a special day because I started to realize that all human beings were related in one big family of mankind, and realizing the joy of this fact made all other considerations unimportant, less than trivial. We were all family, and I was at peace in the wonderment of this one great truth. Because this became so important for me, I had to demonstrate to others and to the world that my belief was strong that family came first and we were all one family. I realized that one of the things that got in the way of our remembering that we were all family was money. Yes, that was it. I had to demonstrate to myself and to the world that money meant nothing to me. Joyfully, I went to my room and gathered all my money together. It could not have been more than a few hundred dollars. I then took it to the living room where some fellows were playing cards. I told them that we were all family members and should love one another, and that money was not important. I began throwing the money I had about the room, saying something like "Take this money. Take all my money. It means nothing."

It was wonderful. We were all family and, for whatever reasons, I had become a very rich "uncle" who could make people happy by giving them everything I had. I was the uncle and everyone in the world was related to me. They were all my cousins, nieces, and nephews. Happiness was here. The world was one. People of all races and religions, of all ages, and of both genders were happily joined in family bonds, and I was "Uncle Fred." It was so wonderful. I had a message that must be shared with all mankind.

Just like Mohammed, I had a message and the message must be shared. There was such joy in my heart as I went from person to person, joyfully greeting each of them as my niece or nephew. I started with the people at the party. Of course, it was Independence Day. And on Independence Day we were all being freed, freed from our blindness. We had not been able to see that we were all one in spirit and in family. How wonderful! I must sing it out to all. I had a mission. I had a job. And it was such a joy to sing out the good news to all.

Before long, of course, I had greeted with joy all of my nieces and nephews at the party. It was now time for me to go forth, spreading joy to all I could find. I went into the street to proclaim to all the great truth that we were all one wonderful family and that we could now be as one in goodness and joy. And I danced and I sang out the great news for all to hear. There were people all around. They were on the sidewalks, they were in the streets, they were in the cars passing by. I must sing, I must dance. All for the wonderment of the spirit of man. I hailed people in cars. Everyone was smiling. Their troubles were leaving them. It was Independence Day at last. People were free. Such wonderful joy.

I had noticed that two of my best friends seemed to be very busy making telephone calls when I had still been back in the house. I knew they must be helping me to spread the joy, but they did seem curiously serious, particularly considering that it was such a joyful day. But I did not mind. I had a world of joyful message to give. Everyone was so happy. Then, as I was joyfully spreading love and happiness, I noticed that one of the cars was not colored like the others. No, it was just black and white. It did not look colorfully joyful like all of the other cars. The black and white car stopped and two policemen got out. They seemed very serious. Clearly, they needed the message very badly. I held up my arms and joyfully yelled, "Nephews, your Uncle Fred is here! Isn't it wonderful! We are all in the family of mankind." The police were very nice, but firm. They suggested that I get in the back of their car. How wonderful it could be that the police were now going to help me, Uncle Fred, spread the joyous message. It certainly seemed appropriate, but somehow something did not seem quite right. But I did not worry. I was still quite confident that joy was here at last and that my mission was a sacred one.

In fact, the police were quite good. In a similar situation in later years, the police were to ask me whether I would prefer to go "to jail or to the booby hatch." But these gentlemen knew exactly where to take me with my message. After a 20-minute ride, during which I saw lots of people to whom I could wave and proclaim the message, we arrived at a place with very big, old buildings. The police asked me to follow them, and one of my friends joined us. He had evidently been following the police in his car. I now realized that I was in a kind of hospital. I was told that I would be talking to a doctor. I came to understand that I had been brought to the Columbus State Hospital. Later I was to learn it was commonly referred to as "the looney bin on the hill, " or just "the hill," by many who were familiar with it.

The physician I talked with was a very serious man. He did not seem to appreciate at all that I had a joyous message. Most people smiled when I gave them my message. But the doctor did not smile. He also had a very thick Spanish accent, and it was a little difficult for me to understand what he was saying. My friend told me that he was sure that everything would be all right. He looked a little sad, but I knew he wanted to get back to the party. Then two men came and told me to follow them. I was a little reluctant to go with them. They seemed to have no reception to my message of joy. They grabbed me by the arms. I went along with them. I knew that I had a mission and nothing could keep me away from my purpose. As the men escorted me, they started laughing, but it did not seem to be a joyful laugh. I began to become a little afraid that they might try to harm me. I didn't really resist them, but I was not going along with them in joy either. They brought me to a ward. On the ward were many "nephews." I began greeting them with joy. I told them that I was

Uncle Fred and that everything would be all right now. Most of my nephews seemed to like me, but for some reason I was placed in a seclusion room before long. I do not know why. The seclusion room was small and I do not remember anything being on the floor. There was a small window about 2 feet by 18 inches that was open to the outside. It had vertical bars on it. The door of the seclusion room had a hole about the size of a half dollar in it, so I could see into the day hall of the ward.

I stayed in the seclusion room for some time. I could see some of my nephews in the day hall. One of them kept goose-stepping back and forth and saying things I could not understand. Most of the others seemed fairly quiet. I yelled to them that it was Independence Day and that I was Uncle Fred. I yelled that we were all of one family and that the time for joy had come. They did not seem to react at all.

Before long I began to become thirsty, and a little later I needed to go to the bathroom. No one let me out of the room. I must have soiled or urinated on myself, because I remember that later, when I was let out of the seclusion room, I was walking about with no clothes on at all. I remember walking naked in front of other patients and both male and female staff members. When I drank the water from the fountain, I remember being told to return to the seclusion room. A staff member told me, "Get back to your room." I told them that I was Uncle Fred and I had a message of joy. They became very firm. They wanted me back in the room. I told them that I was Uncle Fred and that I must be called Uncle Fred or I would not pay any attention to them. Two of the orderlies started coming toward me.

When I was in Japan I had studied karate, and I used to practice it a lot. As the orderlies approached, I went into a karate stance and made it very clear I did not want to be touched. I threw punches toward one of them. I did not hit him, but I must have come close, because he backed off. So did the other one. By now the other patients were beginning to take an interest in my activities. I began to strut back and forth in the day hall. "I am Uncle Fred," I said, "and I am here to spread joy on Independence Day. Hello, my nephews. Your Uncle Fred is here for you now."

The staff was now being reinforced. I remember there being a man in a security uniform and an older lady in a nurse's uniform. She seemed to be the one in charge now. I was encircled by the staff members. They were becoming very insistent that I return to the seclusion room. I was just as insistent that I was Uncle Fred, and that I would only respond if I were referred to by the proper title. The security man looked like he might want to come forward to grab me. I fired a karate jab directly at his eyeballs. He moved back. I strutted some more. Truly,

I was Uncle Fred on a sacred mission, and the other patients could all see that the staff would not be able to keep me from my purpose.

The older nurse finally stepped forward and said to me, "Fred, let's go back to your room." I roared that I was to be called "Uncle Fred." She looked at me in the eyes, thought for a moment, and then said, knowingly, "All right, Uncle Fred, let's go back to your room now."

I went back into the room, and I remember staying there a long time. While I was in the seclusion room, I remember holding the bars on the window and yelling to whoever could hear me below, "I am Uncle Fred. This is Independence Day. I am waving my flag. Hooray for the red, white, and blue. I am Uncle Fred and I am celebrating Independence Day by waving my flag out this window."

Before too long it became dark. I did not sleep. It was occurring to me that the Chinese and Japanese were awake now. If I concentrated in the Chinese and Japanese writing systems that I knew, I could be in tune with that section of the human family that was now awake. I knew many ideographs, and by concentrating on them I would be fulfilling my mission. All night I had the joy of knowing I continued to be at one with the family of man, and I knew that no matter what it might look like, I was fulfilling my mission on this earth.

I remained in the seclusion room a long time. I do not blame the staff for not wanting to let me out again. During the days I could yell out my message to my nephews. But before too long the floor of the room had become a mess. I had urinated and defecated in the room, and it smelled very bad. It smelled so bad that I had thrown up, and the floor of the room was a mix of all three of my bodily products. Once or twice, I had slipped and fallen into the mess on the floor, so I too had become very messy. I had to remain standing with my nose pressed between the bars of the window to the outside. I had to have fresh air. I remember that at least once the door was quickly opened and a tray of food was thrust onto the floor. Some of the food became mixed with the slime on the floor. I was hungry. I was thirsty. My room smelled terrible. But I was still Uncle Fred.

After a long time — I think it may have been as much as 3 days — I was released from the seclusion room. I was cleaned up. I started mingling with the other patients. I told them all that I was their Uncle Fred and I had a message of joy for them. Somehow I felt I could organize these guys. They seemed to need purpose. I always referred to them as "Men." They seemed to like my spirit. One day not long after I was released from the seclusion room, one of the black patients came up to me and asked, very pointedly, if I was the one who called himself "Uncle Fred." I said that I was and that I was very pleased that he called me Uncle Fred. But he did not seem pleased. He was about my height and very stocky, and he was clearly becoming upset. He said his name was Tom. And he wanted to know whether I meant to think of him as an "Uncle Tom" if I was an "Uncle Fred." I was quite taken aback. I did not know what to say. I was clearly disturbing this man. I responded that I did not think of him in that manner at all. I became confused. My metaphor was so joyful. But maybe spreading the joy of the family of man was not going to be quite so easy as I first felt it might be.

For some reason I was reluctant to sign the papers they brought me to sign myself into the hospital. The young attorney smiled a little and said, "We really don't need your signature, you know." A day or so later I was taken before a hearing. There were a few doctors there. They asked me if I had ever been hospitalized before. They asked if I had been in any of these hospitals for a long time. I responded that, yes, I had been in the Bethesda Naval Hospital in Maryland for over 5 months. One of the doctors smiled very broadly, looked at the others in the room, and responded that 5 months was not a very long time at all. That day they determined that I was indeed "an insane person," subject to hospitalization under the laws of the state of Ohio. I was committed to Columbus State Hospital that summer of 1968. I did not stay a long time, maybe only a couple of weeks. The hospital determined that I was a veteran eligible for treatment at the Veterans Administration (VA) Hospital in Chillicothe, about an hour's drive to the south. I spent a longer time in the Chillicothe VA hospital. During the time I was there, I remember that the number eight became very special to me. Everything having to do with the number, eight, took on special meaning. In Chillicothe I was also given psychological tests, and told that I had very good academic skills.

Some time later, when I returned to the large house at 143 Frambes Avenue, the site of the Independence Day Party, everyone was very nice to me. I was not calling them my nephews any more. After a few more months, I learned that at that time (in 1968) it was possible to work as a prison psychologist in Ohio with only a bachelor's degree. My undergraduate degree at Tulane had been in psychology. When I was tested for the position, they gave extra points on the civil service exam to veterans. I did not really need the extra points. Not many people applied for the jobs then.

One question on the application form asked if I had ever been mentally ill. I answered in the affirmative. When I handed the form in, the secretary looked at that answer on the form and asked if the illness had been serious. I responded that I had been a patient in several hospitals, including Columbus State. She shook her head. She said that she was sorry but she would have to speak to someone. She did speak to someone. It was a recently hired master's-level administrator. I do not know exactly what he said or how he said it, but the secretary came back and related that, much to her surprise, she could process the application. I am sure she never knew that the master's-level administrator she had asked had been one of my "nephews" at the Independence Day party a few months before.

I did not really want the job. I could speak Spanish and Japanese reasonably well, and I was trained in international business. I was ready to help American industry raise the living standard of the world. But somehow I also felt that perhaps I had better take this job for a short time, just until I could line something up in the business sector.

It is now 22 years later. I am still working for the state of Ohio. A few years after my third "cosmic adventure" the Department of Mental Hygiene and Corrections split apart, and I transferred to the new Mental Health Department. During these years I have earned a doctorate and become licensed in psychology, and for the past 10 years I have served as the psychology director at Ohio's largest mental hospital. We deliver services to many hundreds of psychiatric patients. I talk with many of them every day. And every day, when I talk with them, I know I am talking to the nieces and nephews of "Uncle Fred." And, just as I had, they are all having their own special "cosmic adventures" of one sort or another.

Addendum: Two days after Earth Day, 1990

I wrote the "recollection" above in about 7 hours last Sunday. I broke down crying several times while writing it. The tears felt good. During other times I found myself singing happy songs. As I had explained initially, I had expected I would be much more "paleological" as I explored my memory banks for what transpired early in July 1968. But use of metaphors actually diminished once I began to tell the story. Two days later now my mind is much more rational, but I know my mind always functions a little differently from others.

HOW PATIENTS EXPERIENCE THE INTERPERSONAL ENVIRONMENT

CHAPTER SEVEN

Patients' Perceptions of Families

Much has been written about the interactions of patients and their families. Most of these writings are by professionals, exploring the etiology and meaning of the symptoms of mental illness through a family prism. More recently, family members have been writing about their feelings and experiences in living with the mental illness of their relatives. Patients' writings about their families, however, are few and sporadic. In some cases, they have to be gleaned from first-person accounts that may have only a few sentences relating to family interactions. Some remember positive aspects, and surprisingly few dwell on negative aspects. The important feature in patients' writings, however, is not the evaluative flavor of their family recollections, but the fact that when they appear they are brief and largely incidental to the emphasis on their inner lives, the first episode, and the history of the evolving illness. This is in sharp contrast to a clinical paradigm that for many years viewed family relationships as the essential building blocks of psychiatric disorder.

It is important to recall some of the older views of family dynamics, because for so many years these theories have determined the ways in which clinicians have treated, educated, and modified the behavior of their patients. Family members' treatment by professionals (or their lack of it) has in turn affected their relationships with their loved ones. As some clinicians have noted (e.g., Arieti, 1981; Terkelsen, 1983), patients' perceptions of their families have to a large extent been informed by the attitudes of mental health professionals. Both the quantity and quality of families' helpfulness have been affected by family members' lack of information about major mental illnesses, which can in large part be attributed to the traditional unwillingness of professionals to educate families or to involve them in the treatment process. The theories developed and utilized in the field, however, can be viewed as reflecting clinicians' own coping strategies in trying to understand and deal with the mysteries of mental illness.

HOW PROFESSIONALS HAVE VIEWED FAMILIES

For many years, the main focus both in the literature and in clinical practice was on exploring the etiology of mental illness through eliciting and analyzing patients' recollections of relationships with their parents, and in particular with their mothers. A review of the literature indicates that mothers continue to be lambasted for a range of sins, including but by no means limited to the creation of major mental illness (Caplan & Hall-McCorquodale, 1985)

Regardless of the content of patients' statements, professionals' interpretations almost invariably cast families in a negative light. Negative comments, according to Arieti (1981), have been accepted at face value and subtly reinforced through clinicians' encouraging nods. In contrast, patients' positive statements about their families have typically been interpreted as examples of repression, rationalization, reaction formation, or other defensive strategies. The defenses are viewed as reflections of deep-rooted cultural taboos against expressing hostility toward one's parents, and more particularly as ways of avoiding an implosion of feelings evoked by traumatic events in one's childhood.

Both in psychodynamic and in family systems theories, there are multiple paradigms to explain how people become mentally ill or how a mental illness is perpetuated by the dysfunctional family's needs for the patient's symptoms. The terms "schizophrenogenic mother," "double bind," "mystification," "marital schism, " "marital skew," "pseudomutuality," and "communications deviance" have all been used as explanatory models for patient–family interactions in schizophrenia. Many researchers have disputed these models through a careful analysis of the empirical literature (Eaton, 1986; Howells & Guirguis, 1985; Parker, 1982) or through failure to confirm earlier findings with rigorously designed replications (Hirsch & Leff, 1975). Arieti (1981), after almost a quarter-century of working with persons with schizophrenia, has stated that 75%–80% of the mothers he has encountered do not remotely fit the descriptions of "schizophrenogenic." Nevertheless, the notion of family pathology persists both in parts of the literature and in clinical case conferences. The current emphasis on the concept of "expressed emotion" (EE), although yielding useful tools for family education, has similarly been perverted by many clinicians into a view of families as pathogenic (Lefley, 1992).

Briefly, EE research differentiates between "high-EE" families (those in which at least one family member expresses hostile criticism or emotional overinvolvement toward the patient) from "low-EE" families (those in which no family member does so). Empirical research indicates that significantly more patients decompensate and return to the hospital from high-EE families (Leff & Vaughn, 1985). The EE researchers emphasize strongly that families do not cause schizophrenia and that high EE may be found in many other environments, including psychiatrists' offices (Vaughn, Snyder, Jones, Freeman, & Falloon, 1984).

Despite some cogent criticisms of the concept of EE and its implications for families (Hatfield et al., 1987) there are some beneficial aspects to the research. High EE in the household is just one example of a range of environmental stressors that can trigger psychophysiological arousal and decompensation in persons with a core biological vulnerability to excessive stimulation, and the EE research joins convergent research findings from other domains in highlighting this vulnerability in a variety of contexts (Lefley, 1987, 1992). High EE is thus to be identified and avoided in settings ranging from day treatment programs to board-and-care homes. The EE research has also been instrumental in supplanting older family systems approaches with family psychoeducation. For the first time, clinicians are offering families information about schizophrenic illnesses, behavior management techniques, and problem-solving strategies (Anderson et al., 1986; Falloon et al., 1984). Finally, the international EE research demonstrates conclusively that the majority of persons with schizophrenia live in low-EE families (Lefley, 1990, 1992). Most families in the world, regardless of the symptomatic or functional characteristics of their ill loved ones, show affectionate support, tolerance, and acceptance. This is an important finding that tends to confound stereotypes of schizophrenogenesis.

MENTAL ILLNESS IN THE FAMILY: GENERAL PROBLEMS AND REACTIONS

There is now a substantial literature that indicates the enormous amount of stress faced by patients' relatives. Briefly, family members encounter both "objective burden" (reality-based problems) and "subjective burden" (emotional distress) in dealing with mental illness. Objective burden includes financial hardships; disruption of household routines; curtailment of social activities; impaired relations with the outside world; and excessive time commitments in negotiating the mental health, medical, and social service systems to obtain needed services. Siblings or younger children in a family often complain of neglect of their needs because attention is focused on the patient. Patients' behaviors are often difficult to tolerate. These may include embarrassing actions in public places, mood swings and unpredictability, property damage, sleep reversal patterns, excessive smoking, and poor personal hygiene. Paranoid ideation, attentional deficits, verbal abuse, and unprovoked assault are some of the behaviors reported by families (Swan & Lavitt, 1986). Families report that it is particularly difficult when a patient refuses to continue taking medication, and the family members fear that she or he will decompensate and force them to seek involuntary commitment (Dearth, Lambenski, Mott, & Pellegrini, 1986; Slater, 1989).

Under these conditions, it would not be unusual for family members to react with the hostility or criticism characteristic of high EE. Yet, in their study of violence in 1156 National Alliance for the Mentally Ill families, Swan and Lavitt (1986) reported that parents avoided confrontation or criticism, and that "walking on eggshells" was their primary response to assaultive behavior. The main coping response of families was to calm and soothe the patients, rather than to distance themselves or to call the police. The authors reported that parents who were able to separate themselves emotionally from the violence and to view the patients as ill showed the highest level of positive adjustment.

Yet this mode of response would appear to reinforce negative behavior by not setting limits. In fact, some commentators have suggested that low EE is inappropriate and counterproductive when a patient's behavior calls out for normal social restraint (Kanter et al., 1987). Kanter (1985) is quite firm in stating that psychiatrically disabled persons, no matter how ill, should be held accountable for their actions. Indeed, the critical question is whether tolerance of antisocial behavior infantilizes persons who, under most conditions, demand and deserve respect for their autonomy. Zan Bockes (1989), a former patient, writes that he has little control over his hallucinations but some control over his thinking and feeling, and "I have much control over my behavior" (p. 42). Siblings, who are closer in age and role expectations, often have less tolerance than parents in holding patients accountable for difficult or embarrassing behaviors.

REACTIONS OF SIBLINGS
AND ADULT CHILDREN

In their first-person accounts, siblings and adult children manifest a range of ambivalent attitudes toward mentally ill loved ones. Their coping strategies are consonant with the nature and intensity of their reactions, which are often related to the family ambience as the illness develops. These interact with their own personality structure and strengths.

Brodoff (1988), describing the "invisible baggage" of growing up with a mentally ill brother, recalls the slowly diverging developmental paths of siblings who were very close as young children. The writer enjoyed school, friends, and activities, while the brother's life became increasingly constricted and friendless. She describes her conscious efforts to distance herself from a "loser" who was increasingly denigrated by teachers and peers, and the guilt engendered by her self-perceived cruelty. She also recalls her thankless attempts to include her brother in social activities, which turned out to be fiascoes because of his provocative behavior. And finally, she recalls resenting the paternal attention to her brother and thinking that the only way to get their attention was for her to become sick also.

The direction of siblings' lives often evolves from these initial attempts to understand and cope with serious mental illness. Many accounts recall resentment and wanting to escape; stigmatization and shame; and problems involving the actual or anticipated loss of friends. There are fears of coinheritance, fears of being "different" like an ill sibling, and fears of inheriting the problem after the parents are gone. Some siblings report becoming overachievers because they felt that had to make up to their parents for the loss of achievement by the other child. But there is also mourning for a premorbid personality once known and loved, as well as feelings of deprivation and loss of the companionship and sharing that might have been expected from a more intact sibling. And there is empathetic grief for the pain of the brother and sister afflicted with mental illness. Some siblings respond to the total situation with rejection and distancing, while others remain loving and supportive (see Brodoff, 1988; Moorman, 1988). Many siblings have banded together in the Siblings and Adult Children Network of the National Alliance for the Mentally Ill, enhancing their coping skills in support groups for persons who share similar experiences.

Lanquetot (1984) describes the conflicted emotions of the daughter of a schizophrenic mother. Her memories of childhood are permeated with feelings of shame, embarrassment, confusion, loss, and even terror of a bizarre and abusive parent. However, in most accounts of adult children (and of siblings as well), there is also an underlying note of love. There are recollections of kindness and devotion when the parent is well, commingling with fear when she or he is ill. A substantial number of the offspring of schizophrenic parents, despite difficult childhoods and relatively high genetic risk, emerge as "invulnerable children" (Anthony & Cohler, 1987). Many siblings and adult children immerse themselves in helping others, including joining the mental health professions.

PATIENTS AND PARENTS:
THE CRITICAL ISSUE OF DEPENDENCY

Previous chapters have dealt with the symptoms of acute psychosis, which bring their own terrors and feelings of unreality. About 25% of patients are able to overcome these and go on with their lives (Torrey, 1988). For the majority of persons with severe and persistent mental illness, however, the main issue is not acute symptoms, but disruption of the normal life cycle. Most trace the onset of their illness to the late teens or early adulthood. For some, this occurs before they have even finished high school; for others, psychotic episodes and hospitalizations interrupt college education or abort beginning careers. For many persons, particularly those with schizophrenia, there is a disruption of the normal socialization process, which results in inability to fulfill expected developmental tasks. This social retardation plagues the afflicted individual and is a major area of disturbance and bewilderment to those around him or her.

Most individuals who have not fulfilled the developmental tasks of late adolescence or young adulthood are still rooted in a conflict of independence and dependency. They want their own jobs, careers, mates, and perhaps children of their own. But they are still dependent on their families of origin for economic sustenance and social outlets. Research indicates that social networks of persons with chronic mental illness are small and dense, and that those who have families tend to depend on their relatives for social interaction (Sullivan & Poertner, 1989). There is constant ambivalence about these roles, and this ambivalence evokes self-hatred and anger. Patients need relief from this internal conflict of simultaneously wanting and fearing independence from their families. It is easy for them to displace their anger onto the perceived source—the parents who love them and are least likely to reject or abandon them.

Reinforcing this dependency conflict is the maladaptive burden of guilt maintained by many parents. Torrey (1988) has pointed out that guilt provides an "illusion of control" (p. 277). If parents are to blame for schizophrenia, then perhaps they can prevent its onset in a younger child or can cure their ill offspring by changing their behavior. Conversely, if schizophrenia is a random biological event, people are helpless to prevent its occurrence. This feeling of helplessness is contrary to our entire cultural ethos, and is one of the reasons why clinicians search for causes and cures in human agency. Parental guilt, however, serves to perpetuate dependency. The suggestion that parents are to blame for, and may be held accountable for, the aversive behavior of their offspring tends to infantilize persons with mental illness by relieving them of responsibility for their own actions.

PATIENTS' NEGATIVE OR CONFLICTED PERCEPTIONS OF FAMILIES

Although there are few negative references in the first-person accounts of former patients, survey responses of the California Well-Being Project (Campbell, 1989a) indicated that 31% felt that their families rarely listened to them and considered what they had to say to be valid or important. An even higher number (38%) did not feel "safe" talking to family members, because it might lead to curtailed activities or treatment demands. At the same time, individual patients tried to apologize for their families: "My family didn't know what to do," or "I don't blame my family. They couldn't see beyond me going back to graduate school. What I was becoming, in their eyes, was a successful psychotic" (quoted in Campbell, 1989a, p. 56).

Although many clients felt that their families contributed to their psychological problems, some had parents who themselves were mentally ill. This led to a chaotic family situation, as in this case:

> I had a hard time dealing with my family; I think partly they may have contributed to some of my problems. . . . My mom had shock treatment. There was a lot of disagreement in the family as to her having problems and how they should have been treated. So I don't think I got a whole lot of support from my family. I don't think they recognized that I was going through some hard times. (Patient quoted in Campbell, 1989a, p. 59)

There is a tendency to dispute parental blame and at the same time to fear the implications of a strictly biological explanation:

> A lot of time family members have been accused of making their kids crazy, or that it's hereditary, or that they were somehow bad parents. Unfortunately, the effect that it has on us as clients is that the answer to a medical problem or a biochemical problem is drugs. (Patient quoted in Campbell, 1989a, p. 59)

PATIENTS' POSITIVE PERCEPTIONS
OF FAMILIES

In defiance of traditional etiological theories, the writings of many former patients recall relatively normal childhoods and good relationships with their parents and siblings. In Chapter 10 of this volume, Esso Leete speaks positively about her family members as she traces her illness history. Many persons with mental illness are well aware of their dependency and disruptive behavior, and feel loving gratitude toward their parents for standing by them.

A particularly salutary coping strategy is to confront the issue of dependency by freeing parents from guilt and convincing them that protecting their children may interfere with recovery. In the following comments, Steve Kersker (1990), a Florida consumer, takes on the role of teacher to the world of "parent friends" in a local Alliance for the Mentally Ill newsletter. Kersker's comments are reprinted here at length because they exemplify so clearly that a person may have a mental illness and at the same time be a well-integrated, sensitive personality in his understanding of himself and others. In these comments, he relieves parents of guilt, while at the same time convincing them that they are doing the best thing for their ill children by letting go of the burden of responsibility.

> I am often saddened when speaking to my parent friends by their unfounded belief that they can help their children avoid the unpleasant limitations of their illnesses. Parents are in no way responsible for the suffering of their children. No one is to blame for the unfortunate transformation of a normal life into a life unimagined. Mania, depression, and schizophrenia are illness that one can usually learn to tolerate and to accept while beginning to develop a meaningful life. In my opinion, one cause of our frequent regressions is our severe dependency. Our illnesses on their onset and our response to our changed selves cause us to regress. We return to the defensive patterns of childhood. We feel helpless. We lose hope of ever resuming control over our lives.
>
> Our parents can not protect us forever. We, your children, have to learn how to assume responsibility for our lives including our illnesses. This is why psychosocial rehabilitation centers exist. Our parents have to learn to distance themselves from us while we learn our limitations. Love must let go in order to let us grow and develop. If you cannot let us go, we can never come back to you. To have us return as your sons and daughters, you have to let us become our own person[s,] and you must accept [those] person[s] no matter what the limitations.
>
> The acceptance of realistic limitations gives us a point to be-

> gin. Recovery starts with reality. Psychosocial rehabilitation pro-
> grams give us an opportunity to develop a life of our own around
> the reality of our particular illness. Recovery from a serious and
> debilitating illness takes time, patience, love and understanding. We
> have to start at the bottom in order to overcome our regressive and
> infantile responses to reality. Parents should not try to block reali-
> ty from us. We have to learn to live with reality, whatever our par-
> ticular reality may turn out to be. (Kersker, 1990, p. 2)

In her letters home, Sylvia Plath (1977) similarly applied the coping strategies of parenting her parent by protecting her from guilt. Plath,
the brilliant young poet who committed suicide at the age of 30, wrote
movingly about her suffering in coping with manic depression. She
even overtly acknowledged the dependency conflict: She wrote to her
mother, "I feel like putting my head on your shoulder and weeping
from sheer homesickness" (p. 69), but "I *will* grow up in jerks, it seems,
so don't take my growing pains too vicariously, dear" (p. 71).

When her mother sought her advice about how to deal with a
friend's son who was deeply depressed, Plath wrote: "He probably feels
something like a hypocrite, as I did—that he is not *worth* the money
and faith his parents have put in him. . . . Show him how much chance
he still has" (p. 145). But she counseled against the value of psychodynamic therapy: "I think psychiatrists are often too busy to devote the right kind of care to this; they . . . blither about father and
mother relationships when some common sense, stern advice about
practical things and simple human intuition can accomplish much"
(p. 145).

Plath's acknowledgement of her deep love and admiration for her
mother permeates many of her letters home. She wrote:

> I associate home with all the self-possession and love which is an
> intrinsic part of my nature and find a great overwhelming pleasure
> in coming back from my travels in the realm of adult independence
> to lay my head in blissful peace and security under my own hospita-
> ble roof. (pp. 72–73)

These words, which are self-affirmative as well as loving, are in stark
contrast to a psychodynamic picture of mental illness as caused by poor
parenting. But they are consonant with what is now known about the
biogenetic substrates of manic depression, and the dependency issues
involved in being mentally ill.

Interestingly, some patients take mental health professionals to
task for abusing their parents. Some clinicians misinterpret this as defensive, while others learn to question the prejudices inculcated in their

earlier professional training. Blaska (1991), a former patient with a bachelor's degree in psychology and a master's degree in counselor education, protests her label of "CMI" ("chronically mentally ill") by referring to mental health professionals as "MHPs." (See also Frederick Frese's use of "CNPs" for "chronically normal persons," Chapter 6, this volume.) Describing an example of CMI identity, Blaska writes:

> During your third hospital stay, one of the MHPs approaches you to inform you that they've asked—demanded—that your parents come in. Today. This afternoon at 1:30. Apparently they've replied that they couldn't. It was the first good planting day and your dad was in the fields. They inform you that they threatened to send you to a big State mental institution, if they didn't come in. You express indignation at their ultimatum and defend your parents. They have six kids. You're one of them, but your father has to put food on the table for eight people. The MHPs seem alarmed at your defense of your parents. (p. 174)

Recounting a later conversation, Blaska states that the MHPs told her that the defense of her father indicated that she felt she was less important than the rest of the family—that she was evidencing low self-esteem by viewing their needs as more important than her own. Although it is difficult to second-guess the meaning and intent of professional communications, one thing is readily apparent: The MHPs were viewing Blaska's defense of her family in purely psychodynamic terms, while she, more knowledgeable about planting time, felt she was defending their economic survival. In insisting on a particular time and place for their meeting, the MHPs seemed to show no concern that they were being indifferent to the reality-based needs of a farm family.

Mark Vonnegut (1975), having undergone numerous treatment modalities under the diagnosis of schizophrenia, wrote to a friend with a similar diagnosis to accept schizophrenia as a biochemical abnormality. Like Plath (1977), Vonnegut counseled against insight-oriented therapy:

> Freud himself said that psychotherapy wasn't of any value in schizophrenia and all subsequent studies have borne him out. . . . A more serious problem with most psychological theories and therapies is that they usually involve placing blame. According to their model, your parents, or your friends, or you yourself, or someone else has screwed up. The fact is, there is no blame. You haven't done anything horribly wrong and neither have your parents or anyone else. (1975, p. 208)

Despite the occasional struggles of mentally ill persons with their families (largely over the question of autonomy), and survey responses indicating that patients often feel unheeded and misunderstood at home (Campbell, 1989a), there are few negative references to families in patients' first-person accounts of their illness. The references, in fact, seem predominantly grateful to families. Part of the recovery process for many patients is learning to see and appreciate their families' contributions rather than to view them as obstructive, or to forgive family members for not having understood the depths of their despair. For many patients, a major part of recovery involves learning how to effect a balance between independence and dependency needs, and to affect the limits of an autonomy that may be too stressful. Self-understanding reinforces the value of interdependence—an acknowledgment by the mentally ill person that he or she may take and give at the same time. In a first-person account of problems of living with schizophrenia (Anonymous, 1989c), a former patient concludes:

> Overall . . . I have good people as friends, and a fine family, and I am not forced into a position of taking on too much independence or of being too dependent. I am a unique and interesting person: I don't always fit in with the world, but I think I add something to it. (p. 5)

SUMMARY AND CONCLUSIONS

Most accounts of patients and families have been written by professionals, and these typically have viewed family relationships as essential building blocks of psychiatric disorder. Patients' writings usually have focused on the psychotic experience or on the patients' interactions with the treatment system, with mentions of families brief and sporadic. Patients' references to family relationships have been more positive than negative, however, with many patients expressing sympathy and remorse because of the pain caused to others by their illness.

We now have a substantial body of research literature that indicates the stress involved when families try to cope with mental illness of a loved one. Family members face objective burden (reality problems) and subjective burden (emotional distress) in trying to deal with the treatment and social service systems, balance competing family needs, and manage their responses to difficult behaviors. Siblings, young children, and adult children living with mental illness in the family often describe psychological consequences related to their particular role relationships.

This chapter has discussed the critical issue of dependency in the relations of parents and their mentally ill adult children. For the majority of persons with severe psychiatric disability, the main issue is not acute symptoms but disruption of the normal life cycle. Persons unable to fulfill normal adult productive roles in society remain rooted in unresolved adolescent conflicts of independence and dependency. We suggest that role ambivalence evokes self-hatred and anger in many persons who simultaneously desire and fear independence from their family support system. Many parents have accepted a maladaptive burden of guilt under the illusion that this will help their child.

Patients' negative or conflicted perceptions of families are revealed in some writings and survey responses. Some persons feel that their families do not validate their needs or have contributed to their psychological problems in the past. Some have parents who were themselves mentally ill and created a chaotic household. Others excuse their families on the grounds that they did not know what to do when the illness became manifest.

Many patients, however, write positively about their families and recall relatively normal childhoods and good relationships with parents and siblings. In their personal accounts, persons with long psychiatric histories frequently express gratitude toward their families for standing by them during years of dependency and disruptive behavior. Some specifically absolve their parents of guilt or defend their families from the misinterpretations of mental health professionals. Psychodynamic models often have interpreted such positive statements as indicating denial, repression, or rationalization. However, patients themselves affirm that their rejection of family blaming and assumption of responsibility for their own recovery are evidence of coping strength. Optimal coping seems to be demonstrated in patients' recognition of their limitations, understanding the contributions they can make to society, and acknowledging an interdependence that allows them to give and take at the same time.

CHAPTER EIGHT

Patients' Perceptions of Professionals and the Service Provider System

We find a number of common threads in patients' accounts of their experiences with the mental health system. Older writings, primarily in book form, are more likely to describe the tumultuous inner world of madness than the external environment (e.g., Kaplan, 1964). In today's literature, most first-person accounts continue this focus on the internal aspects of psychosis, but the writers also describe their transactions with the treatment system into which they were catapulted because of their illnesses. Many former patients, particularly those who suffered involuntary commitment, tend to dwell on the compounded humiliations of incarceration. Others suggest that they achieved neither symptom alleviation nor rehabilitation in the mental health system.

Nevertheless, there are indications throughout the literature that many people feel they have benefited from treatment and from their interactions with particular staff members. Many members of the consumer movement attest to being helped by professionals and remember the concern and devotion of special individuals. Some feel that they might not be alive today if it were not for hospitalization, and many are grateful for psychotropic medications. In this chapter we present some survey findings and direct quotations representing the range of patients' perceptions of mental health service providers, and of the system in which providers work.

PATIENT-STAFF RELATIONSHIPS IN THE HOSPITAL

The early patients' movements, particularly protest groups such as the current National Association of Psychiatric Survivors (formerly the National Association of Mental Patients), were largely based on the premise that the mental health system itself can be a repressive and counter-therapeutic force. Especially in institutional settings, these groups maintain, a message of inadequacy is transmitted through the paternalistic attitudes and behaviors of mental health professionals and the front-line staff members who model their behaviors. The mental hospital is viewed as a place for restricting and dehumanizing mentally ill people rather than as a source of healing. In her recollection of the mental hospital as a "funny farm," Anonymous (1989a) expands on the pejorative term with cogent sarcasm. She describes

> a hospital that is more like a farm—a place where people described as sick are treated like animals; a place where nurses serve as ranch hands, placing feed at regular intervals in tiny paper cups . . . ; where unpredictable human behavior is viewed as "crazy" and where predictable animal behavior is viewed as ideal. (p. 2)

A similar view, but with kinder explanations, is found in the recollections of a former patient who later worked on a psychiatric inpatient unit:

> My illness improved and my doctor got me a job on a psychiatric unit in a general hospital. I spent four years there working among patients as an aide and observing everything, including the staff. The staff was hardworking and dedicated, but I noticed that even among the "enlightened" there are attitudes that will not go away. The staff becomes tired and frustrated with the behavior of the patients and soon adopts negative attitudes about them. This is supported by the technical vocabulary of mental health professionals. Patients are called infantile, regressed, passive dependent, and these terms are used out of the purely scientific technical contexts in which they were originally embedded; but the impression staff gives is that they conclude that the patients are childish and immature. (Barbera, 1982, p. 25)

These attitudes, in turn, translate into functional restrictions on patients' autonomy. One of the most prominent writers to focus on the demeaning and restrictive aspects of hospitalization has been former patient and present-day consumer advocate Judi Chamberlin. According to Chamberlin, "The whole experience of mental hospitalization promotes weakness and dependency. Not only are the lives of patients controlled, but patients are constantly told that such control is for their own good" (1978, p. 6). In contrast to the knowledgeable, competent staff, patients are deemed inadequate, untrustworthy, and in need of supervision. This strips patients of self-esteem and decision-making capabilities: "Patients become unable to trust their own judgment, become indecisive, overly submissive to authority, frightened of the outside world" (1978, p. 6).

In this view, psychiatric hospitalization is not only repressive but intrinsically countertherapeutic, because it takes away the very skills needed for adapting to life outside the institution. Rehabilitation in the community then becomes deflected from its goals of training for a productive life, and instead becomes a mode of restoring the psychological and functional competencies that have been eroded by institutionalization — that is, belief in one's own capabilities and the capacity for making appropriate choices.

RELATIONSHIPS WITH PROFESSIONALS IN THE COMMUNITY

Power and Control Issues

In many community programs, clients show little difference from institutionalized patients in perceiving demeaning messages from professionals. In the California Well-Being Project, a survey of 331 clients in the state system revealed that 57% reported being told that they were resistant, rebellious, or "mentally ill" when they disagreed with the opinions or advice of mental health professionals. Almost 56% felt that mental health professionals only infrequently listened to them or considered what they had to say to be valid or important. Some felt that their rights to privacy had been violated; others felt that professionals punished them for defending their rights (Campbell, 1989a).

In Estroff's (1981) study of the Program for Assertive Community Treatment (PACT) in Madison, Wisconsin — surely one of the most highly esteemed outreach and rehabilitation programs in the country — even this best-case scenario yielded evidence of hierarchical relationships and inequalities of control, based on one's identity as "crazy" or "normal." Although this ethnographic study took place in the early days of a model program that may have made substantial changes since that time, Estroff's description certainly holds true for many programs today:

> In nearly every dimension, normals, both insiders and outsiders, had more control than clients and other crazy people over those aspects of living that attest to independent, positive selfhood. Clients' resources, in particular, were subject to almost total control by normals. . . . During treatment, PACT staff had almost complete control in each area. When there was exchange, it was not equivalent.

Staff had access to information about clients which clients did not have in relation to staff. (1981, p. 185)

Estroff cited Chamberlin's (1978) suggestion that psychiatric patients ultimately concur with evaluations of themselves as "sick" or "incompetent" because they are usually not encouraged to relate to one another in helping roles. Estroff, however, noted that in her interviews with PACT members,

Clients themselves perceived their friends as not giving help when it was needed. My ethnographic data are filled with clients' remarks about one another's craziness and incompetence. The empirical question should be raised as to whether these attitudes can be changed. (1981, p. 187)

This ethnography was done over a decade ago, and in fact Estroff's own research and insights have been instrumental in changing attitudes and expectations of the system with respect to consumers' capabilities. Much has transpired in changing patients' attitudes toward their own capabilities and those of their peers. These developments are discussed in greater detail in Section IV.

Patients' negative feelings about the mental health system focus on other issues beyond the power and control aspects of the provider–patient relationship. Some patients complain of being required to attend day treatment programs that offer little in the way of rehabilitative skills, inadequate vocational training, and indifferent psychiatrists who spend 10 minutes a month in cursorily evaluating their medications. Negative feelings toward psychiatrists are frequently associated with negative feelings toward psychotropic medications.

Attitudes toward Medications

Estroff (1981) interviewed 32 clients taking Prolixin on their attitudes toward the drug. She found that only 3 had a positive attitude; 7 were ambivalent, offering pros and cons; 11 were neutral or indifferent; and 11 were "decidedly and vociferously anti-Prolixin" (p. 97). Among those who were ambivalent, one client listed the following pros and cons:

Pros: 1. Prevention of insidious psychosis; 2. Keeps me from dramatic mood swings, thinking disorganization; 3. Possibly improved reception to therapy.
Cons: 1. Physical manifestations of Prolixins [sic]: (a) increased nervousness, (b) uncontrolled tremors, (c) mood changes . . . ;

2. Physical man[ifestation] from Artane [a drug given to relieve some of the side effects of Prolixin] (a) dryness of mouth, (b) lightness of body causing upset stomach; 3. Difficulty in concentration; 4. Difficulty with excessive nervousness, shuffling feet, and moving digits of hands; 5. All of the above contribute to the feeling of despair, anxiety, and restlessness. (quoted in Estroff, 1981, pp. 91–92)

From the patients' accounts, Estroff (1981) noted the following reasons for aversive feelings toward psychotropic medication: "fears about the drug, resistance to perceived control by others, strong dislike of side effects, and a reluctance to acknowledge the need for psychiatric medication and the existence of psychiatric problems" (p. 97).

Among these reasons, side effects appear to be a particular problem, both because they are physiologically troublesome and because tremors and movement disorders interfere with social and vocational functioning. In the California Well-Being Project, more than half of those taking psychiatric medications reported suffering from side effects — 28% "severe" and 24% "moderate." "However, 54% of those clients surveyed indicated that their doctors or therapists 'seldom' or 'never' inform them of the risks or benefits of their therapy or care plans" (Campbell, 1989a, p. 159).

Divergent Perceptions of Clients and Professionals

The California Well-Being Project also highlights the discrepancy between clients' and professionals' perceptions of issues relating to information, respect for clients, confidentiality, and trust. The professionals who were interviewed portrayed matters in a positive light:

Most professionals report that (1) clients feel safe talking to them about personal matters or their innermost feelings (66% of 103 report "all" or "most of the time"); (2) they inform clients of the benefits or risks of their care plan (63% out of 103 report "all" or "most of the time"); and (3) they personally treat clients with whom they work with courtesy and respect; 100% of 150 professional/caregiver respondents said either "all the time" or "most of the time." (Campbell, 1989a, p. 137)

The clients, as noted earlier, saw things very differently:

Many clients do not feel that: (1) they are fully informed of the benefits or risks of their care plan; (2) they are listened to and con-

sidered to have something valid or important to say; (3) the mental
health system respects their civil and human rights; and (4) they
are safe when talking with professionals about personal matters or
their innermost feelings. (Campbell, 1989a, p. 137)

These revelations seemed to be tied into the clients' feeling that they
did not have free choice in selecting their own therapists, but had to
make do with assigned staff members regardless of rapport or goodness of fit. In the California Well-Being Project as a whole, the following issues appeared to be paramount in patients' perceptions of their
relations with professionals: lack of free choice and informed consent;
hospitalization and involuntary commitment; seclusion and restraint;
misdiagnosis; and psychiatric medications (Campbell, 1989a).

A perusal of the California clients' open-ended answers, however,
indicated that their views were not uniformly negative, as these themes
might suggest; nor did they imply rejection of services. The free-choice
issue suggests that clients would have utilized the service of supportive psychotherapy more willingly if they had been able to choose their
own therapists. For example, one client stated: "I believe that the
therapist–client relationship is a very personal relationship. I wanted
to find someone I could trust" (quoted in Campbell, 1989a, p. 54).
Psychiatric medications were viewed both positively and negatively:
as necessary for control of emotions, but also as producing aversive
side effects. The misdiagnosis issue was closely tied to selecting the
most appropriate and helpful medications.

PATIENTS' POSITIVE FEELINGS TOWARD
SERVICE PROVIDERS AND HOSPITALS

Although there are many justified complaints from clients about their
treatment in the mental health system, a substantial number of present
and former patients acknowledge their own denial and express thank-
fulness for psychiatric intervention at a critical time. In his moving
memoir of suicidal depression, the noted writer William Styron (1990)
even takes his psychiatrist to task for discouraging hospitalization: "In
my case he was wrong; I'm convinced I should have been in the hospital weeks before. For in fact, the hospital was my salvation" (p. 68).
Elsewhere, he states that the hospital "should be shorn of its menac-
ing reputation, should not so often be considered the method of treatment of last resort" (p. 72).

Styron, however, had a relatively brief period of psychosis, and
by his own admission never assumed the identity of a mental patient.

Moreover, he stayed in a private hospital for only 7 weeks. Styron is a well-known professional writer, but many former patients are in fact encouraged to write as a therapeutic measure, and these are the ones most likely to remember fondly the psychotherapists who were their mentors.

Mark Vonnegut (1975) has described his fall into madness and subsequent recovery through a judicious combination of medications and vitamin/dietary therapy. He has kindly feelings toward many of the professionals who helped him, but contempt and anger toward the antipsychiatry movement represented by R. D. Laing. In a letter to a friend evidencing signs of schizophrenia, Vonnegut noted:

> I myself was a Laing–Szasz fan and didn't believe there was really any such thing as schizophrenia. I thought it was just a convenient label for patients whom doctors were confused about . . . The point is that there is overwhelming evidence that there is a very real disease. (1975, p. 207)

In an earlier article, he showed bristling outrage toward Laing's suggestion that schizophrenia is a transcendental growth experience:

> He's said so many nice things about us; we're the only sane members of an insane society, our insights are profound and right on, we're prophetic, courageous explorers of inner space. . . . It would be nice to be able to hang something as destructive and wasteful as schiz [sic] on the alienation and materialism of modern life, to have all that pain be noble and poetic instead of senseless and useless. . . . But what I felt when I found myself staring out of a little hole in the padded cell was betrayal. "I did everything just like you said, and look where I am now, you bastard." (Vonnegut, 1974, p. 90)

Unlike Styron, Vonnegut, and other graduates of relatively short-term stays in private hospitals, many individuals contributing to this literature at present are former mental patients who have suffered years of illness, multiple long-term hospitalizations, and numerous crisis admissions to public-sector hospitals. Many have developed their writing skills and generated their own therapeutic growth through involvement in the consumer movement.

The consumer movement is roughly divided into three attitudinal subgroups: those who are generally hostile toward the mental health system and bitter about their experiences; those who work readily with professionals and incorporate them into their support groups; and those who pursue a middle ground. Data from a national survey of 104 self-help groups found that the majority were middle-ground groups in which partnerships with professionals could occur but were problematic. Less common were radical antipsychiatry groups that eschewed any dealings with professionals, and conservative, propsychiatry groups that welcomed professional partnerships (Emerick, 1990). This survey has been discussed in greater detail in Chapter 2.

Even in the radical consumer movement, however, criticism of hospitals and psychiatrists is not always uniform. Wade Houston, an original editor of *Madness Network News* (affiliated with the Network Against Psychiatric Assault), wrote approvingly of his hospital treatment and described his psychiatrist there as "a good friend" and "very sensitive" (Hudson, 1974). The California Well-Being Project, which was a product of a consumer group, found that among community clients who had been psychiatrically hospitalized, 50% felt that their hospitalizations had been "somewhat" to "very" helpful; 25% felt that hospitalization had been "helpful in some ways" and "harmful in some ways," only 20% found psychiatric hospitalization "very" or "somewhat" harmful (Campbell, 1989a). Since this study was designed and conducted by former patients, these findings pose a serious threat to the impression that mental health consumers are predominantly opposed to psychiatric hospitalization.

Many consumers, moreover, express outrage similar to that expressed by Vonnegut (1974) in contesting the "myth of mental illness" philosophy. Joe Rogers founded the National Mental Health Consumers' Association, the largest of the consumer groups, as a home for ex-patients who did not subscribe to the doctrines of the antipsychiatry movement. Issac and Armat (1990) had several interviews with Rogers:

> In some respects Rogers proved a devastating critic of anti-psychiatry orthodoxies . . . "I was crazy before any psychiatrist met me, so if it's psychiatric oppression they have real good secret ways of doing it." There was nothing romantic, inspiring or wonderful about mental illness, said Rogers. "It is horrifying, terrifying, and destructive to the soul." "Those of us who have suffered from serious illness," said Rogers, "need to speak out against those charlatans in our movement who claim that somehow our pain and our despair can be translated into the language of fairy tales." (p. 223)

Barbara Pilvin (1982) speaks of the terrible, self-defeating damage of denying one's illness:

> Denial . . . can have crippling or even deadly consequences for those who, psychotic or not, and encouraged by adamant adherents of

the absolute right to refuse treatment, decided to end their treatment or refuse to accept it. Denial of the illnesses' existence (by those who aren't psychotic) is, ultimately, a product of stigma, which is what we should be fighting. But there are some well-known psychiatrists . . . and lay advocates . . . who instead waste precious time applauding and even encouraging denial. It's not a medical condition . . . It's just different or antisocial behavior. Really? Take a look at a PET scan series, Dr. Szasz. Three scans, same brain, manic in one, normal and depressed in the others. The differences are striking even to a layperson like me. They should be: the brain could be mine. (p. 22)

In contrast to consumers who equate control with their ability to reject medication—in effect, a denial of illness—Pilvin assertively controls her life by fighting the temptations of denial:

> I will not be crippled or killed by my disease. Even at the time of my first episode I knew instinctively that denial would destroy me. . . . Denial is out of the question. My life is too precious. . . .
>
> With time and growth, acceptance becomes easier. Growth means coming to terms with the conflicts, successes and failures inherent in striving both to accept our world and ourselves. We *can* come to terms with these, with the help of our friends, families, psychiatrists, religious counselors and others, and of our sense of humor, religious beliefs and ethics, professional interests, personal passions. . . . I still resent the disease, for it has caused me indescribable pain. . . . In an odd way, however, I'm thankful for it, for it's made me understand that there are no guarantees in life, that the outcome of my plans may be beyond my control. The only certainty is that without the pills I would die, but that with them . . . I can lead a normal life. (pp. 22–23)

CHAPTER NINE

Community Acceptance
and Self-Perception

Community acceptance is a multifaceted phenomenon. Overall, it is evident that mentally ill persons continue to be stigmatized and depreciated by an unfeeling society. Formerly, however, they were locked up behind walls—largely unseen by, and out of contact with, the public. Now, with the increasing visibility of homeless individuals on the streets, symptomatic but harmless mentally ill people seem to be looked on more kindly than substance abusers and other members of the underclass. Periodically, letters to newspapers will express pity for their plight, or call for mandatory treatment of psychiatrically disabled street people in hospitals so that they do not end up in jail. Although these visible sufferers are avoided and despised, the public still seems to feel some concern regarding their life conditions.

When mentally ill individuals are treated, stabilized, and prepared for community re-entry, however, this does not mean that they are accepted by society. Stigma is the most critical burden suffered by persons with major mental illnesses. Stigma is an objective, everyday phenomenon. The message that mental illnesses are undesirable and that their bearers should be feared and avoided is transmitted in multiple ways—by the mass media, by employers, by neighbors, by former friends, and even by some family members.

In this chapter we discuss some very real consequences of objective stigma. People may have reached a desired level of functioning after successful treatment, often with enormously hard work on their own, and yet find it difficult to get on with their lives because of societal restrictions. Accompanying the reality-based problems posed by objective stigma—difficulties in finding housing, employment, or social outlets—is the subjective suffering that these messages entail. The perception of not being accepted or respected by the community in which one lives, of not being welcome, is certainly a cause of suffering and diminished self-esteem.

As part of the California Well-Being Project, consumer Leonard Kaplan has stated:

> The worst thing that I've found is the self-stigma that has happened to me. As far as my ego is concerned I've been humbled. . . . I don't think it's my fault, but I feel less capable, less competent, less worthwhile than a so-called normal person. Inside I feel less competent because people expect me to be less competent — because I've been in the hospital for so many years. (quoted in Campbell, 1989, p. 45)

Another consumer reinforces this view of stigma as a response to societal expectations. Dylan Abraham (1982) suggests, "Stigma is not the problem of the mentally ill but of society. The stigma is caused not by the illness but the prejudice of society brought about by ignorance of the medical cause of mental illness" (p. 30).

Many consumers seem to be more comfortable than the general public in equating mental and medical illness. Because psychiatric disorders are manifested behaviorally rather than physiologically, people find it difficult to view them in the same category as organic disease. Moreover, despite media coverage of biogenetic research findings, ambiguous messages continue to be transmitted to the public by a professional community in conflict about the biological parameters of mental illnesses and the issues of cause, control, and accountability. It is easier for people to interpret the positive symptoms of schizophrenia, or the agitated behaviors of manic states, as evidence of an illness than it is to see depression, withdrawal, or apathy in the same light. Hallucinations, delusions, grandiosity — hearing voices, talking with God, or identifying oneself as the Queen of England — are consonant with our cultural notions of madness. But when a person sleeps long hours and refuses to communicate, help around the house, or look for a job, this is closer to our cultural notions of laziness and inadequate character. Psychotropic medications can control positive symptoms, but have less of an effect on negative symptoms. This often leads the public, including family members, neighbors, and friends, to assign a moral label to a person showing such symptoms as well as to the behaviors themselves.

Stigma affects persons in every conceivable way: psychologically, economically, and in terms of their quality of life. Esso Leete (1982) suggests that stigma is understood at first hand when

> your college refuses to admit you after discharge because you now have a history of mental illness . . . you are denied a driver's license because you were stupid enough to answer their questionnaire truth-

fully . . . your friends decide they need to develop other friendships
upon learning of your past troubles and treatment. (p. 3)

Any knowledge of their history affects the chance of mentally ill persons to obtain decent housing and employment, regardless of their qualifications.

HOUSING AND EMPLOYMENT

Social prejudice against mental illness has a direct impact on people's lives. For example, Bruce Link (1991) cites a study in Toronto in which researchers responded to all local newspaper advertisements for apartments to rent. In some cases a research team member indicated that she or he was a patient in a mental hospital who would be discharged within a few days and was looking to rent an apartment, whereas in a control condition a call was made to the same landlord with no mention of this. When the status of mental patient was known, only 27% of the apartments were available, as opposed to 83% in the control condition.

A psychiatrist has reported on the difficulties encountered by a group in Minnesota that for 8 years had a residential housing program for former patients in 21 individual homes, duplexes, and apartment buildings:

> Despite our program's being a good neighbor and an unmitigated success, we have had difficulties, basically concerning community acceptance. I have had to file a suit before the Eighth Circuit Court of Appeals to remain in the neighborhood. The community believes that our program is bad for real estate values, that our residents are dangerous, and that we have established a "mental health ghetto." This certainly is not the case. Our residents remain approximately six months, and 80% of them advance to independent living. Furthermore, none of our residents has ever been arrested, let alone charged with any crime against any neighbor or citizen. (Janacek, 1991, p. 16)

In job-seeking and placement, a stigmatizing message is conveyed not only to employers, but sometimes by members of the helping staff. Funding of mental health agencies often depends on the statistics they can provide demonstrating that they have improved clients' ability to care for themselves. The main goal for staff members becomes one of "returning the patient to independent living" by obtaining employment or housing, rather than restoring the client's skill levels or feelings of personal adequacy. Obtaining any kind of job becomes an end in itself, even if it is inappropriate or requires hiding one's disability. A former patient writes:

> I was told by Disability Aptitude Testing not to discuss my illness with employers. At my present job, there is a very nice woman who frequently talks openly about her diabetes, kidney problems, etc., has her pills on her desk, and no one is shocked; she is not fired. If I did the same with my chemical imbalance, I would be out of a job. I am tired of lying about my job history. I would like to say, "I am schizophrenic, I have limitations." (Barbera, 1982, p. 25)

Nevertheless, the counselor's injunction has a basis in reality. A client in California reports, "I never thought in my life it would ever take me four years to find a job with two degrees from an accredited university" (quoted in Campbell, 1989a, p. 40). A client in Wisconsin says, "Restoration through employment sounds good, but many employers will tell a person who is mentally ill that he or she has no skills for the job, and in reality that person does have personal talent and work skills" (Abraham, 1982, p. 30).

The unfortunate results of disclosing one's history have been recounted by a former patient who lost a 4-year job after confiding to her employer that her brief hospitalization had been for psychiatric reasons. In her subsequent months of job seeking, she faced the following dilemma:

> Many job applications would inquire about medical and psychological stability. For example: "Have you ever been medically or psychiatrically hospitalized?" "Are you now [consulting] or have you ever consulted a therapist?" I found myself in a trap. If I were honest, as I naively was in the beginning, most assuredly I would never (and did not) hear from that interviewer again. If I discreetly manipulated my work history and possibly obtained the position, I might risk a future discovery and be liable for automatic termination. (Anonymous, 1989d, pp. 14–15)

In the California Well-Being Project, a survey of the experiences of 331 mental health clients, 41% reported that "all" or "most of the time" they felt treated differently when people discovered they had received mental health services or had a psychiatric diagnosis. One respondent stated:

> If you tell them about your history and apply for a job they won't give you a job. If you tell the landlord about it when you're applying for a room or an apartment they won't give you that apartment.

They generally avoid you once they find out. (quoted in Campbell, 1989b, p. 25)

SOCIETAL RESTRICTIONS: THE CATCH-22 PHENOMENON

Estroff (1981) has written cogently about the double binds built into a mental health system that is largely funded by public monies. Mentally ill persons, dependent on entitlement benefits for survival, are caught in a maze of legislative and bureaucratic regulations that have presumably been enacted to ensure that able-bodied, able-minded people will not steal from the public trough. Thus, as soon as persons with any kind of disability begin to recover functioning, they are penalized for getting better by being threatened with loss of benefits.

The system is predicated on a notion of linear progress in which mentally ill people are expected to follow a straight path of improvement to independent living. The cyclical nature of bipolar illness, and the ups and downs of schizophrenia, are not taken into account; nor are the physical limitations of persons who cannot cope with undue stress and high-demand environments considered. A former patient pairs a suggestion with a critical question:

> The answer may be to rebuild society as a whole, if that were possible. It is obvious that the mentally ill need low stress jobs and these should be provided for them, or if they can't work, they should be entitled to disability. I cannot get disability now because I have demonstrated too much strength. However, what will happen if and when I relapse? (Barbera, 1982, p. 25)

It is ironic and sad that the recovery process of mentally ill persons is accompanied by a growing ability on their part to perceive the actual parameters of stigma. When a patient is highly symptomatic, his or her perceptions are disorganized and filled with delusional content. The "community" is often viewed through a paranoid lens, so that others are perceived as constantly talking about the patient, typically in depreciating ways. As the veil of delusion lifts, the person with mental illness begins to see and hear more clearly the actual content of others' messages. Too often, in the world of reality, the message is indeed depreciating.

INTERNALIZING STIGMA

The coping skills of mentally ill persons are clearly affected by the manner in which they accept, process, and evaluate their illness. Although some are able to distance their personhood from the illness, for others it becomes a core identity (see Estroff, 1989). For many, stigma begins with their first treatment episode. A consumer has said, "Once you walk through the doors of the mental health system, you are a mental patient. The stigma is there. It's too bad, because for most people the mental health system is all that they have" (quoted in Campbell, 1989a, p. 52). Another adds, "Once I crossed that line and had to be hospitalized, I felt very ashamed and like I wasn't like everyone else. I didn't want anyone to know" (quoted in Campbell, 1989a, p. 54).

Bruce Link (1991) suggests that a patient's internalization of societal views of mental illness becomes a self-fulfilling prophecy:

> The more patients feel that people devalue and discriminate against mental patients the more they feel threatened by interactions with others. . . . The uncertainty, tentativeness, and withdrawal that can result may affect performance in the job market, social network ties, and a patient's view of himself/herself. (p. 5)

In his research, Link used a 12-question scale on perceived devaluation and discrimination against mentally ill persons. He found that "the more mental patients expected devaluation and discrimination as measured by this scale, the less likely they are to be employed, to earn a good income and to have robust social support outside their immediate household" (p. 5).

COPING WITH STIGMA:
MALADAPTIVE AND ADAPTIVE STRATEGIES

Persons with a history of mental illness have difficulties meeting strangers and making friends. New acquaintances are typically assessed on the basis of their appearance, dress, and manner of speaking, and particularly in terms of their occupational role and ascribed status in life. Persons with a history of mental illness may appear perfectly normal to a stranger. But unless they have reached a stage of militant self-affirmation, most will become uncomfortable about disclosing their occupational status or background, or revealing in any way that they have a disability. Although in relations with others people are constantly advised to "be yourself," persons with psychiatric histories find it difficult to respond to others on a natural, easy-going basis because they are legitimately unsure of their welcome. Unschooled in deflecting personal questions, they may become guarded, suspicious, and hostile. For most mentally ill persons, interactions with the interpersonal environment are secretive; they are afraid, with good reason, of being rejected, avoided, and condemned.

A major argument among theoreticians has been whether "schizophrenic behavior" is purposive. One argument holds that all symptomatology is functional—that it is both a manifestation of inner conflict and oriented toward evoking a certain response from others. A more parsimonious argument, however, is that the "purposiveness" of much of the behavior of mentally ill persons can be interpreted as a mode of coping with a potentially hostile community environment.

As we have noted briefly in Chapter 2, persons who feel stigmatized and socially devalued begin to develop a battery of defense mechanisms. Some of these defenses are counterproductive, ranging from self-defeating withdrawal on the one hand to hostile confrontation on the other. Ambivalent about their own status, some persons with a psychiatric history vacillate between self-devaluation and projecting their anger onto others. They may act grandiose, not as a symptom of delusion but as a coverup for low self-esteem.

One of the most shattering aspects of the "mentally ill" identity is that such persons almost never can relate to others as simply other human beings; they are identified in their own minds, as well as those of others, as individuals who are "different" and whose difference is negatively rather than positively valued. Some persons respond to this by exaggerating their differentness. Even if they are not currently symptomatic, they may act or dress bizarrely, using theatrical exhibitionism to show that they are unique and interesting individuals. Others may exaggerate their dependency and act childish, seeking indulgence because of their status as persons not in their right minds.

An essential feature of being mentally ill is powerlessness. Throughout most of their illness history, patients report having felt powerless in numerous contexts. Crisis intervention or hospitalization has often involved forcible removal and deprivation of their right to informed consent. In many of their writings and oral reports, people are likely to recall the humiliation and helplessness of incarceration, rather than the psychotic behaviors that necessitated their restraint. Some individuals handle powerlessness through coping strategies that may bring temporary gains but that are essentially maladaptive. One example is manipulation. Patients may learn how to wheedle and coax cigarettes, money, or other desired items from family, staff, or other patients. In the long run, their manipulative success strips them of more adaptive and socially constructive ways of earning what they need.

The common Freudian defense mechanisms—denial, repression, projection, displacement—are found in persons with mental illness as well as in the general population. Denial as a defense mechanism is extremely maladaptive for those who use it to reject medications. Sometimes other, equally maladaptive coping strategies are used to provide an illusion of normality. Provoking anger in others is sometimes a mechanism for validating one's normality. In our culture, it is impermissible to be openly angry at individuals who are so mentally ill that they cannot help what they do; one can be angry only at people who are accountable for their actions. Conversely, some people may provoke angry outbursts and then use their status as mental patients as a shield for provocative behavior.

Almost all of the maladaptive behaviors are used to achieve minimal gains for persons who lack power to achieve them in other ways. In recent years, however, as society has become more knowledgeable about patients' potential and more protective of their rights, the defensive strategies of patients have become more positive and proactive. Some patients are beginning to view their "patienthood" as a learning experience, and have become politically active in pushing for their rights as citizens. The consumer movement is the most constructive way of doing this, since it involves development of organizational and political advocacy skills, mutual sharing and support, and a vehicle for regaining pride and self-affirmation. In the course of these activities, consumers are beginning to fight stigma on numerous fronts, beginning with changing our language.

FIGHTING THE POWER
OF PEJORATIVE LANGUAGE

Many clients are beginning to have less need to hide their status as mental patients. Indeed, early antipsychiatry groups such as the Mental Patients' Liberation Project in New York City, the Mental Patients' Liberation Front in Boston, and of course the National Alliance of Mental Patients, defiantly used this identifier in naming their organizations. The Insane Liberation Front, which originated in Portland, Oregon, and the *Madness Network News* continued this precedent of using pejorative terms with pride. In recent years, however, the National Alliance of Mental Patients has changed its name to the National Association of Psychiatric Survivors, to indicate even more clearly how members identify and evaluate their experiences.

The terms used in the ex-patients' movement were deliberately selected to show how members felt about their relationship to the system. Those who felt like "survivors" obviously had negative views. In contrast, the more moderate National Mental Health Consumers' Association was organized by former patients who acknowledged the validity of mental illness and viewed themselves as users and purchasers of needed services. Rather than viewing the psychiatric establishment as a totally unmitigated evil, they saw their function as one of correcting inequities and exposing and fighting maltreatment.

It is of great interest that in assessing the salience of terms commonly applied to mentally ill people, the California Well-Being Project survey of mental health clients found some distinctions in the pejorative impact of specific labels. Although the majority objected to all labels, some seemed more disparaging than others. Over half of the 331 clients surveyed objected to specific linguistic terms. The percentages objecting to each term were as follows (Campbell, 1989a, p. 53):

"insane"	77%
"crazy"	76%
"wacko"	74%
"mad"	70%
"sick"	67%
"flipped out"	66%
"space cadet"	64%
"disturbed"	61%
"psychiatric inmate"	60%
"mentally ill"	58%
"mental patient"	56%

It is apparent that the three least objectionable terms refer to the respondents' identity as mentally ill persons or as consumers of services ("psychiatric inmate" and "mental patient"), whereas the most objectionable are the cruel metaphors and adjectives of an unfeeling society. Since these words are part of the common lexicon, applied daily without conscious malice, it means that persons with mental illnesses must constantly cringe at terms that equate their condition with the most devalued forms of human behavior.

In recent years the consumer movement has also objected to certain terms used by professionals as well. The term "chronically mentally ill" (CMI) has long been used to refer to a functionally impaired population of persons who have periodic needs for crisis stabilization and hospitalization, and ongoing needs for outpatient care and long-term rehabilitation. Chronicity is usually defined in terms of three criteria—diagnosis, duration, and disability (Bachrach, 1988). Although there seems to be a core group of mentally ill persons throughout the world who meet these three criteria, there is some question as to the effects of cultural variables on their numbers and distribution (Lefley, 1990).

Many consumers object to the term "chronic," which for them

depicts irreversibility and poor prognosis. In deference to this feeling, agencies such as the National Institute of Mental Health have been substituting terms such as "seriously and persistently" or even "severely" mentally ill; these substitutes seem to be more acceptable to the people who must live with these labels. Some consumers prefer the term "psychiatrically disabled" to "mentally ill."

Regardless of the descriptors, many consumers resent being identified as part of any group beginning with "the," particularly groups identified by specific acronyms. Designations such as "the CMI" or "the seriously mentally ill" (SMI) strip people of their identity as individuals. This opposition does not reflect denial of mental illness; rather it is denial of a fused identification in which the illness rather than the person is viewed as primary. Consumers do not object to being called "persons with mental illness." In describing her reaction to one of the major identifiers used in the field, a former patient suggests:

> If we can be called CMIs — chronically mentally ill — then they, the mental health professionals, can be called MHPs. If we must be relegated to a three-letter acronym — and basically stripped of our identity and individuality — then they too can be lumped into one pot. (Blaska, 1991, p. 173)

BUILDING COMMUNITY SUPPORT

We have spoken of many of the stressors psychiatric patients face in attempting to re-enter the community or simply in trying to adapt to a society prejudiced against persons with mental illness. The roots of prejudice go deep. Some of the dynamics involve the fears of many individuals that they too can become mentally ill, or that they can somehow be contaminated by being in the company of someone with a psychiatric diagnosis. There are many myths that provide a rationale for prejudice — for example, that people with mental illnesses are basically lazy or infantile persons who do not want to work or grow up; that mentally ill persons are violent and dangerous; and, overall, that there is a malingering or factitious aspect to these behaviors. It is very difficult for society to accept the notion that the behavioral manifestations of major mental illnesses cannot be controlled by acts of will.

The proliferation of research findings on the biogenetic roots of major psychotic disorders is beginning to have an impact on cultural attitudes. Television programs and newspaper articles on schizophrenia or manic depression graphically demonstrate genetic linkages and neuroimaging evidence of brain dysfunction and brain–behavior correlates. Organizations such as the American Mental Health Fund and the National Alliance for the Mentally Ill have solicited the help of advertising councils, syndicated columnists, and other people and groups to fight stigma in the broadcast and print media. On national television shows, well-known personalities announce their mental illnesses to the world, and describe how psychotropic medications have helped them regain control of their lives.

There are class action suits to force insurance companies to identify major mental illnesses as medical conditions. For clients and society alike, medicalization removes much of the stigma of behavioral deviance. The notion that mental illness reflects weak character, or that it can be controlled voluntarily by pulling oneself together, gives way to a picture of a biologically based condition that can be controlled by proper medications, sympathetic support systems, and a low-stress environment.

What of the stigma that affects clients' potential for obtaining housing and employment? Many programs are combating stigma by educating and involving their communities in rehabilitation. An example of this is Fellowship House, a psychosocial rehabilitation center in Miami, Florida, which is based on the Fountain House model. Since its inception in the early 1970s, the director, Marshall Rubin, has been actively involved in local business and community organizations such as the Rotary Club. Through these contacts, he has developed resources for transitional employment, obtained donations to special projects, and created a generally protective attitude toward the psychosocial rehabilitation center and its members. Businesspeople sponsor fund-raising events, sit on the board of directors of Fellowship House, and make sure that clients will not face discrimination in local stores and restaurants. Ongoing contact with local merchants, police, and the press spreads public education about the functional potential of mentally ill people and ensures that clients, even those with overt symptomatology, will be well treated in the neighborhood. In this process, many community members learn to discard myths about mentally ill people and to become psychologically invested in their rehabilitation.

Fellowship House follows the transitional employment model of training staff members along with clients, so that the agency can ensure that a job will always be filled in the case of absenteeism or rehospitalization. The PACT program in Madison, Wisconsin, has a similar policy of demonstrating to employers the value of hiring persons with an acknowledged history of mental illness. Many small businesses need occasional help, but can only afford part-time employment for minimum wages. Assurance of reliable part-time workers backed up by a state-affiliated agency is of considerable benefit to employers.

With respect to housing, many mental health programs are attractive to landlords because they are willing to guarantee annual leases for supervised or satellite apartments. Clients who receive federal entitlements, Supplementary Security Income or Social Security Disability Insurance, are often more reliable sources of rental revenue than persons holding jobs from which they can be fired. With the proper education and salesmanship, landlords can be taught to welcome rather than to discriminate against persons with a history of mental illness.

Families, of course, provide a major source of community support. Many family members are obtaining education about mental illness, resources, and problem-solving strategies from their local affiliates of the Alliance for the Mentally Ill. These affiliates are involved in public education and antistigma campaigns, political advocacy for services and research, and mutual support. Part of the Alliance for the Mentally Ill's initiative is to educate professionals about families' needs as caregivers and support systems for their clients. Many professional training programs are beginning to incorporate collaborative models for working with families in their curricula (Lefley & Johnson, 1990). Hospitals and community mental health centers are now beginning to offer programs that provide information about major psychotic disorders, medications and their side effects, and behavior management techniques.

In this section on the interpersonal environment, we have moved from the terrifying aspects of psychosis to the ignominy of the status of mental patient—from the internal world to the harsh realities of the external world. Community acceptance has a clear impact on self-acceptance, but the reverse may also be the case. In combating the prejudice against their condition, mentally ill persons may become their own best champions.

The strengths of mentally ill persons themselves may provide the most significant resource for changing community attitudes. We have spoken throughout this book about the extremely important role of consumer groups in building skills, self-esteem, and mutual support. Knowledgeable and articulate consumers are beginning to come into public view as members of mental health planning bodies and the governing boards of clinical facilities. Applying the knowledge gained from their experiences, they are beginning to have an impact on the mental health policies that affect their lives. Former patients participate in clinical training, educating current and future clinicians about the visible potential of persons with histories of severe psychotic episodes and multiple hospitalizations. In the final analysis, consumer self-support, advocacy, and educational outreach may be the most important mechanisms for combating both external and internal stigma.

SUMMARY

This chapter deals primarily with the problems faced by mentally ill persons in community living. These persons must deal with objective consequences of social stigma, ranging from difficulties in obtaining employment, housing, insurance, licenses, and the like to the loss of old friends. Moreover, because legislators and planners have inadequate understanding of psychiatric disorders, the system itself militates against job and housing stability. Persons with major mental illnesses, who are subject to cyclical swings or unpredictable periods of regression, are victims of an entitlement system that is predicated on notions of linear progress to independent living.

Former patients report that they have to lie to obtain housing and jobs, and that they are even advised to do this by helping professionals. First-person accounts of the unfortunate consequences of telling the truth about one's psychiatric history highlight the dilemma of persons trying to retain their integrity and at the same time make a successful community re-entry.

In the process, social stigma becomes translated into subjective or internalized stigma. For some patients, a new, depreciated identity begins with the first hospitalization. For others, the recovery process is ironically accompanied by a clearer vision of society's sanctions and prejudices against former mental patients. People develop a variety of coping strategies, some adaptive and many maladaptive. In interactions with strangers, most mentally ill persons have to be cautious about revealing their histories; they are afraid, with good reason, of being rejected, avoided, and condemned. Some become secretive and withdrawn. Others use manipulative or provocative behavior as maladaptive ways of asserting control.

But many former patients are beginning to develop a variety of positive coping strategies for asserting control. An important effort is fighting pejorative language in the public lexicon. A large consumer survey indicated that people are more comfortable with linguistic terms that relate to their status as mental patients than with cruel terms and metaphors that equate their condition with the most devalued forms of human behavior.

Consumers also consider pejorative, and have been instrumental in changing, certain terms used by mental health professionals. In recent years the consumer movement has objected to the term "chronic," which to them connotes irreversibility and negative prognosis. They have also objected to being lumped under any group beginning with "the," which strips them of identity as individuals, and have insisted on "person language" (e.g., changing "the seriously mentally ill" to "persons with serious mental illnesses"). This has influenced many professionals, as well as the National Institute of Mental Health, to use more acceptable terminology.

Various efforts to combat stigma at the national level are described. Well-known personalities have revealed their histories of mental illness and their ability to control their lives with proper medication. Demonstrations of the biogenetic basis of most major mental illnesses in educational campaigns and national media programs tend to destigmatize these poorly understood disorders and to give hope to their victims.

The final section has dealt with mechanisms for building community support and acceptance at the local as well as the national level. We have reported in some detail on a psychosocial rehabilitation program that has built linkages with local businesses, police, and merchants. Businesspeople are involved in governance, fund raising, and public education on behalf of the program, and community members are not only educated but given a psychological investment in the rehabilitation of mentally ill people. Incentives that make it attractive to employ or rent to mentally ill people have also been discussed.

Families serve as support systems for mentally ill persons, and there is a growing trend for clinical programs as well as local Alliance for the Mentally Ill groups to offer opportunities for family education, advocacy, and mutual support (Lefley & Johnson, 1990). Finally, the role of consumers themselves in changing community attitudes is critical. Increasingly involved in mental health systems planning, advisory and governance boards, and even in professional training, consumers now have an opportunity both to exercise some control over the events that shape their lives, and to change community attitudes about their capabilities. In the final analysis, we feel that through their educational, self-help, and advocacy efforts, consumer organizations may provide the best mechanism for changing both external and internal stigma.

CHAPTER TEN

The Interpersonal Environment
A Consumer's Personal Recollection

ESSO LEETE

Coping with schizophrenia and building a productive and satisfying life for myself have taken me 25 years. My unique interpersonal environment has had a significant effect on my progress, as well as on the full-blown expression of this disease in my midteenage years. Let me begin by putting my life in context, beginning when I was a child and leading to the first signs of my illness. I would like you to recognize as you read this that mine is not a particularly unusual story. I was neither prodigy nor idiot, pampered nor abused. Being a fairly average child did not halt schizophrenia from laying its icy hands on my shoulders and turning me away from the world at large.

During my treatment period over the last 25 years, my interpersonal environment has changed. It has shifted many times among the community at large, school peers, family members, psychiatrists, social workers, and other patients. It is clear to me now that a supportive, accepting, and loving relationship with others — my interpersonal environment — has been the key element in my recovery from this major mental illness.

MY EARLY HISTORY AND
THE BEGINNINGS OF MY ILLNESS

I was the first-born in a family of three siblings and had two younger sisters, Carol and Sue. My father was in the Army and we were obliged to move every 2 or 3 years, including twice to Germany. This pattern was perhaps the most traumatic circumstance in my life; I sorely missed the predictable schools, familiar houses, and consistent friendships that others enjoyed. I remember being fairly shy, but not what I would call really withdrawn as a child. I was an excellent student and put most of my energy into school work and some sports. Changing schools so often put me at a disadvantage, and for this reason I felt great pressure to work harder than my fellow students; there were many times, in fact, when I labored over extra credit reports for various subjects, even though I already had achieved an A in the class.

I had a good relationship with my parents and my two sisters. There were, of course, the usual sibling rivalries and jealousies, and disagreements with my parents over the usual "rights" and "responsibilities." When I was in my senior year of high school, we moved from Germany back to the United States, and my father retired to Virginia. Suddenly I had to begin at a new school, make new friends, and adjust to a new city and even country. It was during this last year of high school that I first became ill. It was at this time that I began to sleep more, to have nightmares, and to be consumed with an intense anger toward everyone. I could not explain it, and indeed I did not understand it. I became very agitated and would run away, and my angry outbursts would often lead to my throwing objects. I could no longer control my impulses. I sensed that something terrible was happening to me, but I felt helpless to discuss it or to do anything to alleviate my suffering.

Except for participation in sports, I had always been more comfortable by myself, and in my senior year I became increasingly withdrawn and sullen. I felt alienated and lonely. Everyone was so distant from me; there seemed to be a huge gap between me and the rest of the world, including my family. I got to the point where I watched dispassionately as my two younger sisters matured, dated, shopped, and shaped their lives, while I seemed stuck in a totally different dimension. I did not then think about what was happening to me, for I was oblivious to it at this point, but looking back now I realize some of the changes I was going through. My family, on the other hand, apparently denied the whole process, no doubt desperately wanting to believe that it was just a "phase" that I was going through. My irritability led to more arguments with my parents. I wanted to discuss what I was reading in school—Greek tragedies and Plato. I could feel my brain changing with this new horizon, and I wanted to talk to everyone about these matters. Actually, I was probably obsessed with these readings and ideas.

I finished my last year of high school successfully, achieving good grades, but I was not doing well emotionally. I continued to withdraw from my family and classmates, in whose presence I felt self-conscious and awkward. Something told me I was different, and I just naturally tried to avoid people. I sat in the corner by myself in classes, or would otherwise physically remove myself from others as much as I could. I felt less uncomfortable if I wore my long heavy winter coat everywhere; I wore it for security, and I don't think I took it off that entire year. When classmates or teachers spoke to me, I often could not reply or mumbled some response without looking up at them. Although I was an honor student, I felt stupid and inferior.

About this time my family was making plans for my college education. I was terrified. It was very scary for me to think about going to a new city, even state, where I would not know anyone. I had no idea what to expect. Although I did not know what would be asked of me, I was sure I would not be able to perform whatever it was. I felt as though I were being abandoned, punished by being sent away into an unfamiliar land. Yet I put up a fairly good front, knowing that this move was expected of me, and made my plans with my parents step by step. I had some offers for scholarships based on my good grades, but all of these colleges were out of state. I knew, therefore, that I would be leaving; I also knew that I was unprepared, but I tried not to think about this.

I arrived at college in Florida and did the best I could in my new surroundings. I knew no one there and felt isolated from the rest of my peers, who seemed to be making friends and adjusting to college quite well. I was also easily disoriented, and it took me quite some time to memorize the location of classroom buildings. I would go to class and sit in the back, wanting to be as invisible as I could, already realizing that my ability to concentrate and absorb the lessons was greatly diminished. Repetitively, almost compulsively, I would draw face after face of Van Gogh. This seemed to comfort me. In addition, often I would write poetry, which flowed from me without effort or conscious thought. I did not always understand my poems, but this did not concern me at all. It was just something I had to do, probably to alleviate my anxiety about my new surroundings.

For my semester German project, I decided to read a German novella in its original and interpret it by writing a comprehensive paper on it, also in German. I got the project approved by my German teacher and began immediately. I read the novella probably two or three times. I saw fantastic symbolism in the book, with deep meanings both for myself personally and for the world, and I knew it was no coincidence that I had chosen this particular piece of literature. I began writing my paper. I began to dream about the book and became obsessed with it. Every detail held secret meanings, and I wrote furiously to capture them all.

Soon after I had completed this project, I experienced my first real psychotic episode. It was evening and I was walking along the beach near my college in Florida. Suddenly my perceptions shifted. The intensifying wind became an omen of something terrible. I could feel it becoming stronger and stronger; I was sure it was going to capture me and sweep me away with it. Nearby trees bent threateningly toward me and tumbleweeds chased me. I became very frightened and began to run. However, though I knew I was running, I was making no progress. I seemed suspended in space and time. I panicked, but with effort pointed myself in the direction of my dormitory and continued on.

Finally, after what seemed like hours, I arrived back at my dormitory. By this time I was hearing voices and responding to them. I was confused, disoriented, and frightened, and remained in a different reality. I made it back to my dorm room, where my roommate realized something was terribly wrong and comforted me as best she could. Although I was hearing voices for the first time, I truly believed that everyone must hear voices. I thought nothing of it and was absolutely unconcerned. Over the next few weeks I continued to have auditory hallucinations, still not comprehending that I was out of touch with reality as others knew it. That reality had given way to the multiple realities with which I would now live.

I had no close friends in college, and few professors who I felt really knew me. However, I did feel close to my German teacher, and it was he who ultimately asked to see me in his office and stated that he was very concerned about me. I had no idea what he was talking about. It did not occur to me that he had noticed my decompensation. He asked me if I would speak to the school psychologist. I had no idea why he wanted me to do this or what it would accomplish, but I tried to please this professor by going. I spoke to the psychologist for about 45 minutes and was given a referral for a visit to a psychiatrist in town. I still was totally ignorant of any problems.

After a boring time in his waiting room, the psychiatrist finally introduced himself to me and asked me to follow him to another room. I explained the sequence of events that had brought me to his office, and he asked me many questions, without giving me much feedback or response to my answers. I patiently waited for him to finish his interview. At the end of the session, he simply held out his hand, said goodbye, and thanked me for coming to see him. As if it were my idea! It seemed kind of pointless, really, but I said goodbye and quickly left his office.

I returned to my dormitory and college life. It was an existence of loneliness and isolation. I had a total of two friends, one of whom pressured me to do drugs, the second of whom pressured me to get married (regardless of the fact that we barely knew each other). I turned both offers down and withdrew further into myself. I waited for letters from home, which rarely materialized. Looking back on this time, I feel now that had I been able to establish even a couple of close, trusting relationships with my fellow students, I might have been able to deal with these changes in me more realistically.

I still do not know exactly what transpired from that point on. I myself thought nothing more of it and went back to sleeping in my clothes, going to class (late), and not eating or showering. One day soon after, however, I returned to my dorm room and was surprised to find my father there, my bags packed and waiting at the door. Someone must have notified him of my condition, for he had come to take me away. This did not feel like support; it felt like treason. I was shocked and angry, yet could not pull myself together enough even to object. He told me we were going to take an airplane home for a while. I don't even think I asked why; perhaps I already knew. At any rate, I compliantly followed him out and got on the plane with him. There I remember furiously writing a lengthy treatise on some great (but incomprehensible) subject that seemed very meaningful to me at the time. We did not speak or look at each other; I was barely aware of my father sitting next to me on the flight home.

We arrived, and I began my first in a long succession of psychiatric hospitalizations. I had now become aware of what was happening to me, and I became extremely frightened. I had no idea what would await me in the hospital, and I was terrified of the unknown. My parents tried to console, comfort, and reassure me, but I remained suspicious. I have now been hospitalized approximately 15 times, the longest hospitalization lasting a year; have had twice as many doctors; and have received numerous medications and treatments, including insulin coma therapy and electroshock. Over the years I have reluctantly become an expert in the area of my illness. I have absorbed my losses and been surprised at my victories. I have learned coping mechanisms to deal with my mental illness, and I have tried to pass my information along to others, nevertheless realizing that each of us must ultimately fight our own battle with our own individual demons.

THE IMPORTANCE OF
THE INTERPERSONAL ENVIRONMENT

Perhaps our environment, both internal and external, holds the key to our recovery, even though the illness itself may be a biochemical abnormality resulting from a genetic predisposition. In the most concrete way, our environment can be either relaxing or stressful. For many individuals with a mental illness, we must learn to go through life experiencing our surroundings with a greater intensity than others do. Sounds are louder, lights brighter, color more vibrant. These stimuli are distracting and confusing for us, and we are unable to filter their impact to lessen their effect. In addition, I believe we are more sensitive in an interpersonal sense as well. I have noticed that others like myself are easily able to pick up emotional nonverbal cues and feelings that may be "hidden."

Interpersonal relationships are extremely important both in terms of personal support and in terms of treatment that works. I know that when I first became ill, my parents were told that I would be in and out of institutions the rest of my life and that I would never lead a normal life. This was the framework within which they tried to offer me support and assistance. Although my family was just as ignorant of mental illness as most other families in the 1960s, they did show support as I struggled with it. I'm sure my sisters were embarrassed about my behavior, and possibly angry about the attention I was getting, yet they never abandoned me. It is true that I could not talk to any of my family members because I was too paranoid and angry, but a part of me was aware that they were there for me if I could ever turn to them. This seemed futile to me, however, because I knew that my family would not understand. This is why family education is so invaluable.

In addition, being able to develop an attitude of trust and friendship with my therapists (and others) has aided me immeasurably with my task of recovery. I have been in many systems and been exposed to various kinds of therapy, but none of it was ever effective without there first being a solid, trusting relationship between myself and these professionals.

An Example of a Negative Treatment Environment

However, for purposes of contrast, before I elaborate on my successes, let me briefly describe some dubious approaches to my care during one hospitalization that I found particularly destructive (Leete, 1987b). At this facility I was banned from group therapy, my food was monitored, my time was strictly regulated, and my roommates were removed from my room and thus from my "negative influence." Toward the end of my hospitalization, I was placed in seclusion and restraints every day. I was forbidden to cross a red line painted on the floor, much less leave the unit. Not surprisingly, I did not improve, as such power struggles and automatic limit setting are rarely therapeutic. The more I was ostracized and punished, the angrier I became and the more I rebelled. Slowly my desperation turned to resignation and hopelessness. To make matters worse, even my private psychiatrist would not speak to me. Although he dutifully came to see me about twice a week (presumably in order to collect insurance payments), he completely stopped talking to me after the first couple of sessions. Not only was his "silent treatment" not helpful, but it contributed substantially to my feelings of despair. It was the epitome of an interpersonal relationship that was destructive to me as a person and thus to my recovery.

The prevalent attitude during previous treatment (especially inpatient hospitalizations) had ranged from condescending pessimism to utter hopelessness. This negative stereotype of our prognosis for recovery, held by many professionals today and embodied in pejorative terms such as "chronically mentally ill," is very demoralizing and destructive to those of us struggling with a mental illness. We deserve better than to be labeled treatment failures and dismissed. If we are "chronic," it is mainly because mental health professionals have failed in their attempts to treat us, which is the inevitable outcome of such a set of negative expectations.

An Example of a Positive Treatment Environment

Although over the years I have received in various settings treatment that was beneficial, I would like to specifically describe the psychosocial rehab program of a community facility that embodied many of the positive aspects crucial to a good program (Leete, 1988). Please note that although I am referring here specifically to Community Care in Denver, other facilities and individuals shared some of these healthy attitudes and contributed to my recovery. At Community Care the program was structured and supervised, yet I did not feel imprisoned and at the mercy of an arbitrary staff. I sensed that the treatment team genuinely cared about me, and therefore I did not feel an ongoing need to test limits. Unlike the hospital staff, the residential treatment team did not assume authoritarian, confrontational postures, which result inevitably in power struggles. Residents were accepted and always treated with respect, and thereby we clients gained in self-respect. Interactions were nonthreatening; we always knew that the staff was on our side.

We believed in the staff because they believed in us, an important discovery. Staff members perceived the residents as first and foremost human beings, and they were available to us for assistance in overcoming the problems in our lives. There was a strong orientation toward success, and an expectation from the beginning that we would all leave and become independent through the continuing process of building on our individual strengths. To help us with this, treatment focused on our healthy and adaptive aspects rather than our deficits. We learned to make the most of our assets through specific problem-solving techniques and daily living skills. To my amazement, I discovered that I did have some strengths on which to build my future, and that there were coping strategies I could learn to manage my disorder and my life more effectively.

My input into treatment was encouraged. The residential treatment team considered me a partner in the recovery process rather than a less knowledgeable inferior, and this increased my self-esteem and promoted my personal growth. The staff did not approach my treatment with a negatively biased view of what I could accomplish. Instead, they believed in my potential, and I began to develop confidence in myself. A real sense of ownership in the program and in my improvement was fostered, and gradually I became aware that I was my greatest asset. Too often, psychiatric hospitals had engendered or exacerbated feelings of dependency and low self-esteem. After several hospitalizations, I had begun to feel hopeless about the future and about my having any meaningful part in the world. The mutual fear experienced by myself and various hospital staffs was replaced by mutual acceptance at Community Care. In addition, medication was used solely as an adjunct in the recovery process, not as a "chemical restraint."

Psychotherapy, both individual and group, has also been an important component of my treatment. Because major mental illness has such a profound impact on all aspects of one's life, I feel that therapy is crucial to explore these areas and to discover ways of successfully coping with the social and personal obstacles raised by such a psychiatric disorder. The combination of psychotherapy and psychosocial rehabilitation can help us with acceptance of our mental illness by helping us to understand the roles of medications, social services, vocational endeavors, residential options, and interpersonal relationships in the management of our symptoms.

As a result of my developing confidence in myself and realistic trust in others, I was able to grow. The prejudice I had encountered was supplanted by an emerging understanding of me as a person, and pity became respect. The flexibility of the program to address and meet my individual needs, recognizing my interests and capabilities, enabled me to work forward with the knowledge that a predictable, consistent, and caring support system was available for me should I need it. Because I knew that support would be ongoing, even when I was officially out of the program, I did not feel anxious or threatened in my attempts at independence.

These characteristics of this residential community-based program are not limited to such an environment. The attitudes of the treatment staff discussed above can be displayed by others as well—family and friends in addition to professional people—and can aid us in our attempts at compensation. Yet even in spite of successful programs like Community Care, we rarely hear recovery mentioned as a possibility for psychiatric patients. Professionals continue to measure our progress with concepts such as "consent," "cooperate," and "comply" instead of "choose," insinuating that we have no control over our illnesses. We can exercise some control over our disorders, and we clients can and should be active agents in managing our own illnesses, as well as partners in the design and implementation of our own treatment. The patient is most familiar with his or her disease and has not only a valid point of view, but an expert point of view.

Let me briefly summarize what helped me in my own recovery process during my stay at Community Care. Finding professionals who recognized and respected my differences and individual needs was crucial to my recovery. I found acceptance and reassurance more helpful than confrontation. Development of coping strategies and social skills enabled me to successfully overcome symptoms and reintegrate with my community (Leete, 1987a). Vocational skills led me to employment. Continuing support and encouragement for my efforts gave me the strength and faith in myself to battle against my disabilities, minimize my vulnerabilities, and work effectively with my individual assets. Being treated with compassion and respect—as an individual with strengths and weaknesses, instead of a mental patient who could never improve—was important. Hope is crucial to recovery, for our despair disables us far more than our disease ever could.

We must confront our disorders with courage and struggle with our symptoms persistently, never viewing relapse as a permanent defeat and always acknowledging remission as a hard-earned victory. In order to meet the challenge of our illness, we must change the image of who we are and who we can become. The paradox remains, however, that only by learning to accept our limitations can we begin to discover our own unique possibilities.

Interpersonal Relationships:
Guidelines for Family Members

Interpersonal relationships serve to aid all of us in overcoming hurdles and enjoying satisfying lives. Our families' positive attitude and support are often crucial to our healthy sense of self and potential, and should complement those of professionals (Leete, 1987). Many persons with mental illness live at home and are cared for by their relatives, and everyone feels increased stress. The family, however, can either contribute to a relapse or be an important factor in the wellness of the individual. This is because interpersonal relationships—that with the family often being the longest, most intimate, and most consistent one—are critical to one's well-being. Although families do not cause mental illness, relapse can be triggered by the family situation, just as it can potentially be arrested or prevented. A consistent, supportive, and honest home environment, in addition to any formal treatment, is crucial to minimize relapse.

I have tried to foster and nurture this type of interpersonal environment in my present family, both for my own sake and in order to develop interpersonal relationships there. I have gone from being simply a daughter to being a wife and a stepmother to my husband's adolescent daughter, Jennifer. Making this transition into a responsible mature adult has been difficult but extremely rewarding. I have been able to offer my husband and stepdaughter love. In addition, this relationship has forced me to become a positive role model for Jenny, a task I try never to forget.

I still struggle daily with my mental illness and the stigma that surrounds it. I have found through the years that in order to effectively combat this, it is imperative for me to learn my own strengths and weaknesses. Developing coping mechanisms is the difference between functioning well and functioning poorly—for everyone, families and professionals included. It is important to encourage those of us with a mental illness to develop our individual skills—coping skills, interpersonal and social skills, leisure-time and work skills—for skills are the best predictor of success, not diagnosis. Family education can also be useful in the long-term management of mental disorders. The following are some guidelines I have put together for family members that may be helpful in this regard:

Above all, be sensitive to our needs and differences and respect them. Give us your continuing support and encouragement. We may need almost constant reminders of love and caring, an ongoing show of faith. Recognize the role of stress, the family, and medications in both the relapse process and restabilization. Involve us in learning about this. Encourage us to participate in understanding the illness by documenting our problems and the treatment, and to look at what happened, why, the effectiveness of the intervention, and what we would like to try next time. Attempt to recognize the early signs of relapse and to know your and our own limits in dealing with the illness. Include us in decision making that centers around possible ways to ameliorate the stressor or mitigate against its effect. Discuss these various options with us.

Be nonjudgmental. Do not embarrass or ridicule us. Eliminate disparaging remarks, criticizing only constructively, with love and understanding. Be patient. Do not shout, threaten, or intimidate. Whenever possible, avoid guilt and hard feelings. Try not to deny or reverse previous responses, plans, or promises. Do not be arbitrary. Explain unexpected changes simply and directly. Comply with requests that are reasonable. Avoid physically or verbally "cornering" us; this includes "hovering." Set and enforce limits if necessary, but do not lose tenderness and compassion.

Recognize both our idiosyncratic thinking and the fact that we may not have the same communication style or skill as you do. First of all, try to minimize distractions during conversations. Be aware of surrounding stimuli and move to a different area if necessary. Communicate clearly and concisely. Avoid ambiguity. Explain what you are saying and why in concrete terms. Speak slowly, in short sentences if necessary. Give the information in small portions. Begin your answers with either "yes" or "no," then elaborate; otherwise your point may be missed. When we are speaking, try not to interrupt. This can be very confusing and frustrating. We're fighting hard enough to speak without being forced to stop and begin again, often on a tenuously held train of thought.

Be sincere and honest. Do not argue or react to us with sarcasm. We are often extremely sensitive. It is fine to disagree or to clarify your point of view, but please do not discount our thoughts or feelings. Indeed, let us ventilate them. Consider that we may have a different perspective, not that we are simply delusional or psychotic. Take what we say seriously. Do not be condescending. Realize that many times we accomplish reality testing with our remarks to you, and we need the assurance of your calm, caring, logical feedback. Be sure to ask us for our input and feelings. Give honest, constructive feedback. Verbally and behaviorally reward our efforts. Treat us with respect, courtesy, and compassion.

Keep your emotional distance, but reiterate positive feelings for us. Do not smother with control or constant suggestions; encourage us to do all we can. Build on small successes. Have and demonstrate confidence in us and our abilities, but encourage us to ask for help whenever necessary. Find a role for us in the family other than being the "sick" member. Focus on our strengths. Do not "institutionalize" us at home. Foster a sense of independence, and rescue only in a real emergency. Provide a family atmosphere that supports improvement of the illness and accepts us, no matter what. Work with us to control symptoms.

Accept that many times we have a real need for seclusion and withdrawal from our environment. I have found it an invaluable means of getting the distance I need from something that was becoming overwhelming. Do not take our withdrawal from you personally. A private place (a bedroom, for example) may be our sanctuary from stress. This "time out" can be used constructively to cope with our symptoms.

Have realistic expectations. Expect good and bad times, and make the most of the good. Set realistic goals together and work toward them together. Do not be devastated by the illness or transmit this hopeless attitude to us. Focus on our strengths as we find ways to overcome vulnerabilities and to help ourselves.

WORKING TOWARD RECOVERY: NEEDS AND GOALS

Sadly, for years I had expected someone else to "fix" me. However, I finally realized, after many clinical disappointments, that this task fell to me alone and that no one else could really make me better. I approached this task very seriously, conscientiously working to get my life back together. For the first time, I then felt ready to take responsibility for myself, including management of my illness, and I feel it was at this point that my recovery really began.

It is important to strive to increase the community's acceptance of those of us with mental illness as well. We need to be recognized as human beings, and as such our right to privacy, confidentiality, and independence must be acknowledged. I am here today to tell you that "mental patients" do have the potential to be self-sufficient and lead autonomous lives. We can responsibly exercise our rights as individuals. When integrated into the community, we can learn skills, work productively, and contribute to society. Too often mental health clients like myself have felt alienated and rejected, vulnerable and powerless, discounted and defeated.

To overcome these negative feelings and our resulting sense of impotence, empowerment is crucial, giving us the strength and confidence to individually and collectively make choices and control our own lives. No longer do we feel powerless: forced into treatment, coerced into power struggles with authorities, and administered therapy that others have determined to be in our best interest. We are changing the image of who we are and who we can become. We are learning to rely on ourselves. We are becoming empowered.

Yet recovery is often never even mentioned as a possibility; there is a profound silence when we ask if we will ever be all right. We are filled with feelings of disgrace and worthlessness as we are continually bounced from hospital to hospital, transferred from doctor to doctor, switched from one medication to another, and thrown into one living situation after another. The only consistent messages we get from others are that we are hopelessly inferior, that we are incapable of functioning successfully, that we cannot be independent, that we will never get well. One reason we experience stigma from the community is that our professionals share this negative perception and resulting prejudices. The seriously mentally ill are seen as beyond repair and hopeless, and for this reason not worth expending much energy on in terms of treatment. This is not true. We clients must defeat our own inner stigma and attack the mistaken views of the public (and professionals) regarding the mentally ill and put them in perspective.

One approach toward gaining this perspective on stigma is through client support groups. A peer-run mutual support group is an effective interpersonal environment in terms of both self-confidence and self-discovery (Leete, 1988). Self-help groups offer each other member support and encouragement, friendship, and hope for the future. We as primary consumers need to meet socially with others who have experienced what we have, to exchange information about coping skills, and to take responsibility for ourselves, because mental patients are a rather esoteric group. We have been ostracized from society, yet we need a group to which we can belong and contribute. Even more importantly, we must meet with others like us in order to see at first hand what we have accomplished and what we can achieve. We will draw strength and hope from each other in this way. We have all suffered, and many have overcome their illness and the stigma surrounding this. To do this, we have had to change the image of who we are and who we can become, first for ourselves and then for the public. It is not easy; it is not quick. The realization that it can be done is one of the most useful aspects of any support group.

Success will never be realized if it cannot be imagined. A peer-run support group can help us understand our disease, and we can learn to function in spite of it by successfully compensating for our disabilities. A support group can give us the personal strength and commitment to overcome the stigma, prejudice, discrimination, and rejection we have experienced, and to reclaim our personal validity, our dignity as individuals, and our autonomy. Here each member is accepted and affirmed, valued and validated. And we can accomplish this with pride, in a group founded by us, shared equally among us, sustained by us, and enriched by us.

Even with these qualitative improvements, life with a psychiatric diagnosis is difficult. I can talk, but I may not be heard. I can make suggestions, but they may not be taken seriously. I can voice my thoughts, but they may be seen as delusions. I can recite experiences, but they may be interpreted as fantasies. To be a patient or even an ex-client is to be discounted. Our label is a reality that never leaves us; it gradually shapes an identity that is hard to shed. Yet it is crucial that both primary consumers and the public at large change the image of the mentally ill. We must ensure that we are seen as people, perceived as worthwhile individuals, and treated as such. We must dedicate ourselves to improving our self-esteem and to achieving a satisfactory life.

Yet too many times our efforts to cope go unnoticed or are seen as symptoms themselves. If others understood us better, perhaps they would be more tolerant. We did not choose to be ill, but we can choose to deal with it and learn to live with it. By learning to modulate stress, we will manage our illness more effectively, thus endowing ourselves with an ongoing sense of mastery and control. I find that my vulnerability to stress, anxiety, and accompanying symptoms decreases as I gain more control of my own life (Leete, 1989).

What makes life valuable for those of us with mental illness and enriches our lives? Exactly what is necessary for other people. We need to feel wanted, accepted, and loved. We need to be productive. We need leisure pursuits that gratify us. We need support from friends and family and a sense of stability in our environment. We need to be accepted by and welcomed into our communities. We need to feel a part of the human race, to have friends. We need to give and receive love. Our need for high-quality and satisfying lives is no different from anyone else's. Sadly, many of us are struggling so hard to meet basic needs that we have little time or energy to devote to these pursuits, leaving us outcasts from our society and personally dejected.

The development of coping mechanisms will help ensure that we mental health consumers are able to meet our basic needs and to fill our lives with hope, productivity, personal satisfaction, and self-respect as worthwhile human beings. The mental health system can assist us both by providing services to meet these basic needs and by working with us to assure a productive and satisfying life. We can achieve high-quality lives of inner harmony by meeting our expectations, realizing our goals, and focusing on our ideals. Warm human contact and companionship, as well as general social recognition, can contribute to our success in these endeavors.

Independence and free choice make life valuable for us mental health clients, as they do for others. Growth toward this autonomy will enrich our lives with a sense of accomplishment and pride, and we can build on these positive feelings. Within stimulating and exciting lives, however, we need security in our environment, both external and intraphysic. We must develop confidence in ourselves and become comfortable with our identities as capable persons in charge of our own lives.

Obviously, we mental health clients do not want to be rejected and ostracized; we need to be accepted and welcomed for our contributions. We do not want to be stigmatized; we must be respected. We do not want to be discounted; we need to be valued as human beings. We do not want to be dealt with in an authoritarian manner; we should be included in all aspects of our treatment. We do not want to be assigned low expectations; we should have hope for attaining elevated but realistic goals. We do not want to be treated in a rigid system of care; we need to be engaged in flexible and individualized treatment. We do not want to have information hoarded and kept from us; we must participate in mutual information sharing with our service providers. As is true of everyone else, we mental health consumers need support, friendship, understanding, compassion, acceptance, tolerance, love, and hope.

Those of us with a psychiatric disability can recover if given the chance. And we have a right to recovery. If we periodically fail in our efforts to achieve this, then let us fail. But we must be given the opportunity to succeed as well. Don't let the mental health system fail us by its entrenched and hopeless view of our potential for recovery, thus further stereotyping the mentally ill and incorrectly convincing us of the futility of our situation. Instead, we must all learn that with rewarding interpersonal contact we clients can change, that we can contribute, and that we can recover.

HOW PATIENTS EXPERIENCE THE RECOVERY PROCESS

CHAPTER ELEVEN

Events Leading
to Recovery

It is difficult to define "recovery" in serious mental illnesses. Traditionally in medicine we have equated "recovery" with "cure" but in mental disorders we do not ordinarily assume that there is a cure. Although improvement in functioning is often noted, we do not have agreed-upon standards of improvement by which to measure progress. For some people, having a job or getting off medications is a symbol of recovery, but these are not attainable goals for many with major mental illnesses (Estroff, 1989).

Autobiographies of patients indicate that they often use the word "recovery," but they mean quite different things by the word. Daniel Link, in Chapter 14 of this book, speaks of recovery from a major mental illness. For him the symbol was a report card that indicated top marks in the first five university courses he had taken. However, he speaks of many intermediate steps along the way: his first attempts to sort out reality from psychosis, his decision to pursue recovery single-mindedly, and his enrollment in a psychosocial program, among others. Link believes that there has been too little research to enable us to understand the dynamics of recovery. Billions of dollars are being spent to ameliorate symptoms, but few resources are focused on the recovery process.

Feldman (1974) has devoted considerable time to the study of a range of chronic illnesses. What he has learned has relevance for the understanding of chronic mental illnesses as well. Few patients with chronic disorders, he noted, return to their premorbid state; therefore, it becomes important to focus on "psychological recovery," or the human aspects of the illness. He advises doctors to include in the management of chronic illnesses a consideration of the social, economic, and behavior complications as well. Of special importance is the kind of response that the person makes to the effects of the illness on his or her life. "Readaptation," he feels, is probably a more useful concept

131

than "recovery": "Readaption demands the reorganization and acceptance of self so that there is meaning and purpose to living that tran-
scends the limitations imposed by the illness" (Feldman, 1974, p. 290).

This leads us back to the theoretical framework of stress, coping, and adaptation outlined in Chapter 2 of this book. We present
this point of view again here as a framework for thinking about the
recovery process.

STRESS, COPING, AND ADAPTATION

Inherent in the concept of coping and adaptation is the belief that all
living systems do more than just maintain themselves. They actively
struggle to surmount difficulties, and they strive to survive physically
and psychologically. They either attempt to adapt to their environment or they try to change it.

This never-ending struggle to adapt and survive in a meaningful
way comes through again and again in patients' stories. Even when
patients seem withdrawn and uninvolved, they may be, as Esso Leete
(1982) has said, actively fighting "internal terrors and external realities" (p. 5) to keep their emotional balance and social composure in
a world they cannot always translate.

Adaptation is probably never an end state that can be achieved
once and for all. Rather, it is a process in which a person continually
attempts to maximize the fit between his or her needs and the environment. Sometimes the adaptation is a psychological one, in which the
person alters attitudes and expectations to fit the requirements of the
situation. White (1974) stresses the frequent need for compromise and
possibly resignation. Events occur that require the person to give in,
relinquish things he or she would have liked, and change directions.
People may sometimes have no choice, he says, but to accept the permanent impoverishment of their lives and try to make the best of it.
At other times adaptation calls for delaying, retreating, regrouping,
abandoning untenable situations, and trying new approaches.

The theorists of coping and adaptation insist that there is an appropriate role for psychological defense in coping with difficult situations. What matters is whether the defense mechanism used facilitates
coping and adaptation (Mechanic, 1974). Monat and Lazarus (1977)
use the term "palliative modes of coping" to refer to kinds of thoughts
or actions used to relieve the emotional impact of stress. There are
the defense mechanisms of denial or diversion of attention, which are
traditionally viewed as pathological or maladaptive, but which can serve
a positive function in reducing stress. George (1974) likewise believes

that classical ego-defense mechanisms can be used constructively in dealing with difficult situations. Such defense mechanisms as withdrawal, denial, and projection need not preclude eventual adaptation; they may help a person maintain psychological equilibrium in order to direct his or her skills and energies to meet a demanding situation.

Although psychological adjustment plays an important role in helping people adapt to external demands, increasing attention is also being given to the importance of knowledge and skills. The field of psychosocial rehabilitation has emerged in the past decade to help people learn how to cope with symptoms and manage their illnesses, develop interpersonal skills, and cope with the demands of everyday living. Strauss (1989a) urges professionals to pay attention to the coping strategies that patients use, as well as to their symptomatology. A more concerted effort needs to be made to separate primary illness mechanisms from coping mechanisms. A person's primary illness may be thought disorder, and hallucinations and delusions may be efforts to cope with this disability. More effectively separating coping mechanisms from illness may make it possible to isolate the characteristics of the illness itself and to understand the person's efforts at healing.

Strauss believes that we need more longitudinal studies in order to begin seeing the patterns in a person's life. He finds that the study of these patterns reveals considerable discontinuity over time. One of the patterns frequently observed is modest improvement followed by a long plateau, which Strauss calls "woodshedding." After what seems to be an excessively long period of no change, patients improve and reach a higher level of functioning. The assumption is that during this quiescent period, subtle activity is occurring that makes it possible to take on more complex tasks.

Another pattern frequently noted by Strauss is that of periods of organization followed by patterns of disorganization with eventual reorganization. This reflects his hypothesis in which coping and illness are closely intertwined. A behavior begun as coping becomes more and more maladaptive until significant disorganization opens the way for new coping strategies. The person will be seen as getting worse or more ill during the period of disorganization, but important changes may occur in attitudes, perception, and meaning—changes that make it possible for him or her to reach higher levels of adjustment.

Strauss's work illustrates the usefulness of a coping and adaptation framework in examining the process of recovery for the common observation that recovery is not a process of gradual and continual improvement over time. Rather, it indicates that adaptation and readaptation go on all the time and that things are not always what they seem.

What appears to be a setback may turn out to be adaptive in the long run.

PATIENTS' PERCEPTIONS OF FACTORS IN RECOVERY

When patients reflect on recovery, they tend to focus on factors or events in their lives that they feel resulted in significant change for them. These factors vary considerably in patients' autobiographical accounts. In this section, we discuss some that have made a strong impression on us.

Acceptance

Frequently patients have said that their willingness to accept the illness was a crucial beginning for them. For Dorothy Minor (1989), this was certainly true:

> My greatest step toward mental health was the acceptance of my illness. The first few years I tried to pretend it was not here. I did not want to believe I was sick, falling to the false logic of medication. Instead of thinking "I am sick; therefore I need medication," I thought, "I am taking medication; therefore I am sick, and if I stop taking medicine, I will be well." (p. 7)

Beverly Cikalo (personal communication, January 16, 1991) said that her first reaction to being diagnosed with schizophrenia was disbelief. Although her family was relieved to find a label for all the trouble she was having, she was not. She continues to feel quite ambivalent about it:

> Seven years later I still deal with my label of schizophrenia daily. I am reminded of my diagnosis twice a day when I take my medication and every week when I get my injection. These days most of my friends are also members of the "mentally ill" category. . . . Friends and family who stood by me often treat me with tender hooks [sic] which only serves to remind me of my chronic illness. What I really *want* . . . is for me to be well . . . and [I wish] that life would be normal. I hate this illness because of what it has done to me and I'm at a loss as to how I can cope with these feelings. What else can I say?

Upon further reflection, Cikalo concludes that her life is not all bad. She has fallen in love and married, and has seen a lot of dedication and caring on the part of professionals. She has improved over time, and with the help of medications she leads a relatively normal life.

In Chapter 14, Daniel Link relates in some detail his gradual awareness that the delusional world in which he had lived for 10 years was not the reality shared by his friends. He sought diligently to return to the reality he knew before his illness. There followed a period of intense emotional upheaval in which grief, rage, and regret enveloped him. Out of this struggle came a single-mindedness of purpose in directing his own recovery, which led to successful academic achievement, marriage, and employment.

In our experience, most families and professionals feel strongly that it is necessary and sufficient for getting better that a person accept a "mental illness" label. Actually, significant differences of opinion are arising in regard to this foregone conclusion. The controversy has been well summarized by Warner, Taylor, Powers, and Hyman (1989) in a recent article. One current theory suggests that a person labeled "mentally ill" may become locked into abnormal patterns because of the way others view and respond to him or her. The result is a poor image that limits the person's capacity for self-control and perpetuates symptomatic behavior (Warner et al., 1989).

Strauss and Carpenter (1981) have indicated that some degree of insight is necessary for effective control over the course of the illness. McGlashan et al. (1975) argue for the importance of acceptance and integration of the illness experience into the patient's ongoing life. The alternative path of failing to confront the reality or "sealing over" the experience, they feel, may have a less positive outcome. In conclusion, however, the authors grant that sealing over may be adaptive for some: "Patients may well have an optimal adaptive style," they say, "which is facilitated by some and impeded by other treatment approaches" (p. 1272).

Responsibility

Feldman (1974) notes that there is a tendency for patients with chronic illnesses to feel that they are victims of impersonal forces operating upon them beyond their comprehension and control. This tendency is especially strong in the case of those with chronic mental illnesses, as we have noted in earlier chapters. Improved functioning, Feldman argues, requires a redefinition of the problem that diminishes the sense of being a victim of forces and that increases the sense of control; he calls this a transition from an identity of being "sick" to one of being "different." This transition usually involves a period of denial and mourning before the past can be relinquished and the future considered. The primary role of the professional is to help the person toward feelings of freedom and choice and of being responsible. Feldman writes:

> To discover a new meaning in the face of the dissolution of the old meaning, to accept the differences imposed by the illness, and to still maintain one's dignity and worth is the essence of the transition from sick to different. When one has accomplished this, there is no need for illness as a primary life style. (1974, p. 289)

Patients providing first-person accounts have related various philosophical ways of coming to terms with their dilemma. Stephen Weiner (1982) has dealt with the unfairness of having mental illness by noting that life is not fair, although it is unfair in different ways to different people. He has decided to accept his condition "without completely giving in to it" (p. 10). But in accepting the illness, he eschews bravado as a means of coping: "Bravado is an almost inevitable reaction to pain and humiliation," he writes. "It is easier to pretend to oneself that the pain and humiliation never existed." But this tactic is a form of denial of the "almost heroic reality that the strength to endure and overcome had to arise as a strategic reaction to an unchosen, unforeseen misfortune" (1987, p. 6).

Zan Bockes (1989) reminds us that life puts various limitations on all people. However, freedom to make choices always exists within these limitations. For him, life is worthwhile in spite of the limitations imposed by a serious mental illness. Barbara Pilvin (1982) tells how she has come to terms with the way that mental illness has compromised her goals in life: It "made me understand that there are no guarantees in life, that the outcome of my plans may be beyond my control" (p. 23).

Hope

Without hope, people could not get better, but it was difficult for patients to identify the source of hope. Esso Leete (1987b; see also Chapter 10, this volume) has identified ways in which families and professionals can play a part in maintaining hope. She suggests that they encourage the setting of realistic goals. She entreats them not to be devastated by the illness and not to transmit a hopeless attitude to ill persons. Such persons will not strive if the effort seems futile.

In a recent *Psychosocial Rehabilitation Journal* article, Patricia Deegan (1988), once a victim of a serious mental illness and now a clinical psychologist, takes the reader on a painful psychological journey originating in hopelessness and despair and triumphing eventually in transcendence and hope. Deegan's companion on this painful odyssey was a paraplegic friend:

> The weeks passed us by but we did not get better. It became harder and harder to believe we would ever be the same again. What initially had seemed like a fleeting bad dream transformed into a deepening nightmare from which we could not escape. We felt like ships floating on a black sea with no course or bearings. . . . All of us who have experienced catastrophic illness and disability know this experience of anguish and despair. It is living in darkness without hope, without a past or future. It is self pity. It is hatred of everything that is good and life giving. It is rage turned inward. (p. 13)

Deegan (1988) goes on to say that for a while giving up and surrendering completely to despair and anguish seemed to be a solution for her and her friends. But eventually, in some unknown way, "the small and fragile flame of hope and courage illuminated the darkness of our despair" (p. 14). They were aware that even when they gave up, people who loved them did not:

> They did not abandon us. They were powerless to change us and they could not make us better. They could not climb this mountain for us but they were willing to suffer with us. They did not overpower us with their optimistic plans for our futures but they remained hopeful despite the odds. Their love for us was like a constant invitation, calling us forth to be something more than all of this self-pity and despair. The miracle was that gradually the paralyzed man and I began to hear and respond to this loving initiation. (p. 14)

We have begun this chapter by raising the question of what "recovery" in serious mental illness is. Deegan has many thoughts about that. She says that recovery does not come in a flash at some point in time. Recovery does not mean cure. Recovery is a process, and hope is the turning point, which must be followed by a willingness to act. Recovery does not refer to absence of pain or struggle; it marks a transition from anguish to suffering. The difference, she believes, is that anguish is futile pain suffered without hope, pain that leads nowhere. When Deegan and her disabled friend became hopeful, anguish was transformed into true suffering and the knowledge that this pain was leading forward into a new future.

Support

Patricia Deegan found that the wise love and support of others were significant factors in her recovery. Many other patient statements carry a similar message. The Canadian Mental Health Association (1985), in a booklet entitled *Listening,* one of several in a series called *Building a Framework for Support for People with Severe Mental Disabilities,* notes that the patient sample the association interviewed was deeply concerned about friends and supports. As one woman said, "I mean, you need someone to believe in you 'cause you don't believe in yourself" (p. 27). Another said:

> What you need is to have a lot of support, even at the beginning. You just need someone to help you get through the rough spots. . . . Here, they're pushing for you to be independent and on your own, but at the same time, they're supporting you. If something happens that you can't handle, they're here. (p. 27)

Comments during the interviews, according to the association reflected the patients' personal struggle between dependence and independence. They often hesitated to ask friends, neighbors, or coworkers for help or support because they believed that their requests would be rejected.

For emotional support, these former patients tended to mention informal relationships and friends most often. But some indicated that making friends was difficult:

> It would be good [to have a couple of friends]. And people my own age, too. . . . Yes, it's important to have common interests for sure. You can't always spot the loneliness. There are so many ways of covering it up. (p. 29)

> My experiences have recently been so different, and other people's lives are so busy, that it is difficult to develop a shared reality with people so you don't feel alienated and out of touch. (p. 29)

Involvement in the "former-patient subculture" seemed to be an important coping strategy. Self-help groups and drop-in centers were means for sharing with others who had similar experiences. Several former patients found that assisting others helped build relationships and a more positive sense of self (Canadian Mental Health Association, 1985).

Barbara Fenwick (personal communication, December 21, 1990) says that support was the most important factor in her recovery. A friend visited and encouraged her when she was in the hospital, and the friend left her own family and moved in with her for a month when she was released. The friend nudged her on and would not let her give up. "She would set me straight," according to Fenwick, "and she wouldn't let others feel sorry for me." Fenwick acknowledges that her friend had a lot of power over her, for she threatened to withdraw her support "if I did not work at getting better."

Fenwick's friend devised a 7-year plan of rehabilitation using all the resources she could muster, with 2 years of the plan being completed before the friend moved away with her family. Fenwick's husband then retired from the Navy so that he could carry out the program. Local mental health resources were utilized, and so were other community resources, such as adult education. Fenwick's husband has insisted that she take English courses so that she will learn to concentrate and communicate better. He goes with her to classes.

Fenwick says that her own goals are still undefined, although she sometimes feels that she might like to become an occupational therapist. She thinks that she hesitates in setting goals for fear the she cannot achieve them. But she trusts her friend and husband to help her. She has come a long way from the time when she was in hospitals more than she was out, and when she actively sought self-destruction in every way possible—even requesting electric shock treatments because she thought they would kill her.

After many years of a most painful struggle with schizophrenia, Marcia Lovejoy (1989) found her salvation in a democratically run halfway house where choices were real, and in the support that its members gave to one another:

> The halfway house changed my life. First of all, I discovered that some of the staff members had once been clients in the program. That one single fact gave me hope. For the first time I saw proof that a program could help someone, that is was possible to regain control over one's life and become independent. (p. 26)

Theorists in stress and coping believe that social supports do play a major role in modifying or mitigating the deleterious effects of stress on people. The presence or absence of support is seen as a key factor in the outcome of a crisis. Caplan (1974) defines "social support systems" as attachments between and among individuals that promote mastery of emotions, offer guidance, provide feedback, validate identity, and foster competence. People help by sharing tasks, supplying extra resources, and giving practical advice and information.

Although the beneficial effects of support networks have generally been acknowledged, there is less understanding about how these supports actually influence psychological adjustment. One point of view says that social supports have a direct effect on adjustment; the other says that social supports mediate the relationship between stress and adjustment (i.e., they serve as a buffer for the individual). The latter model seems to be getting more attention in research at this time (Hatfield, 1987b).

Professional Services

Chapter 8 has discussed patients' perceptions of the helpfulness of mental health professionals. That chapter may be usefully reviewed at this point. Clearly, patients believe that the quality of mental health services can be critical to their recovery.

Patricia Deegan (1988) believed that "we can create environments in which the recovery process can be nurtured like a tender and precious seedling" (p. 15). Rehabilitation programs must respect the importance of small beginnings and the likelihood of failures as well as successes. Deegan feels that many programs are too linear and define failure in absolute terms, thus working against the process of recovery. To nurture growth, they must be structured so as to embrace the approach–avoid and try–fail dynamics that are the essence of recovery. The fact that each person's journey of recovery is unique necessitates a wide variety of rehabilitation options.

Deegan feels that too often rehabilitation programs are based on traditional American values—rugged individualism, competition, personal achievement, and self-sufficiency—and as such are invitations to failure for many. An alternative type of program (or even an alternative life style), in which cooperation and mutual support are central, should be available as an option. We must recognize how much disabled people can give to each other—hope, strength, and mutual sharing.

Finally, staff attitudes are fundamental in shaping rehabilitation environments. "Us–them" attitudes often prevail; "staff" and "clients" are deemed worlds apart. Deegan believes that for an environment to be nurturing, the rigid world separating the "world of the disabled" and the "world of the normal" must be torn down. Staff members, too, have suffered anguish and experienced personal tragedy in their lives. This should make it possible for them to understand the woundedness and vulnerability of people in rehabilitation programs.

Mental Health Services

The role of various treatment approaches and rehabilitation services in recovery does not come through clearly in the patient statements we have examined. Patients tend to talk more about strategies they have used and the role of support and hope in achieving recovery than about the role of specific treatment facilities or rehabilitation services. However, two of the consumers who have written chapters in this book, Esso Lette and Daniel Link, found that a good psychosocial program was very important in their development.

Esso Leete (Chapter 10) stresses the importance of interpersonal relationships in treatments that work. No therapy worked for her until she found a therapist she liked and trusted; this took time and occurred only after many failures. She reports many examples of staff combativeness and rejection. She was given the "silent treatment" by psychiatrists and was ostracized and punished by staff members; attitudes ranged from "condescending pessimism" to "utter hopelessness." Leete also describes the kind of psychosocial treatment service that eventually worked for her. There she found that residents were accepted and treated with respect. Staff members believed in each person's capacity for growth and focused on the healthy, adaptive aspects of his or her personality. The client was considered a partner in the recovery process.

Daniel Link (Chapter 14) says he was fortunate to have the resources of Independence Center, a psychosocial program in St. Louis, Missouri, to help him in his recovery. Through this agency an apartment and transitional employment placements were made available. His self-esteem was enhanced by his assignment to handle members' financial accounts, and eventually he was assisted in securing state vocational rehabilitation funds to pursue a degree in social work.

SUMMARY AND IMPLICATIONS

In this chapter we have tried to learn from patients' accounts the factors that they feel played a part in recovery. Recovery, for the purposes of this chapter and this book, is not defined as achieving a cure; rather, it is thought to be a process of adaptation at increasingly higher levels of personal satisfaction and interpersonal functioning. It involves finding meaning and purpose to life that goes beyond the limitations imposed by the disorder.

Authorities in the field do not believe that recovery occurs at a given moment in time, but rather that is it a long, involved process of forward movements, regressions, and plateaus. Longitudinal studies are needed to chart the recovery process and to identify common pattern or themes among patients. We need to know to what extent there is inherent in each patient, however deeply buried, a natural tendency to struggle for meaningful survival. Then we need to know what kinds of environments are most supportive of these efforts and what kinds of interventions may prove effective at key points along the way. Current efforts at intervention are based on a very primitive understanding of the individual and the healing process.

The concepts of "acceptance" and "control," which have emerged in this and earlier chapters and are used by researchers and patients alike, appear to have considerable usefulness in understanding the recovery process. It is generally believed that acceptance of the illness is a necessary condition for recovery and that its polar opposite, denial, is a serious hindrance. In addition, it is thought that the patient must have some sense of control over the course of the illness in order to use treatment to good effect.

We know little about the way a sense of control develops in individuals. Are there attitudes and ways of relating to patients that influence them in one direction or another? Are there approaches in psychotherapy or rehabilitation that can effectively shift a patient away from a sense of being a victim of his or her symptoms and toward a sense of control over them? Patients' statements suggest that it is easy to err in regard to how much independence, initiative, or responsibility to expect. Some appreciated the clinicians who told them in a straightforward manner that getting better was up to them, that they should take charge of their lives. Others felt misunderstood or abandoned when given similar suggestions.

The concept of "acceptance" is also fraught with difficulty. What we usually mean by "acceptance" is that the patient verbalizes an acceptance of the label "mental illness." We assume that the patient has the same understanding of the term as the professional has. This may or may not be true. There may be different definitions of what is wrong in the person's life, and therefore differences in what is actually being accepted. There are patients who acknowledge that something is wrong, but who refuse the label "mental illness." They may define their problem as "nervousness," "hypersensitivity," or "having a breakdown" and yet cooperate with treatment. There are still others who admit to mental illness long enough to seek treatment and then block out further thoughts about it. They show little curiosity about their psychotic experience, do not want to talk about it, refuse to associate with other mentally ill people, and make every effort to find a place in the regular community. There may be a number of avenues toward adequate adjustment to these illnesses.

CHAPTER TWELVE

Developing an Acceptable Identity and New Purposes in Life

With treatment, the more acute phases of mental illness tend to remit, and more energy is available for patients to orient themselves to the external world. But Harris and Bergman (1984), directors of a case management agency in Washington, D.C., have observed that getting better can be a mixed blessing. Patients find themselves caught between the familiar patient world, which is well defined, and the nonpatient world, which is replete with ambiguity. They are frightened about the future, but they cannot return to the past. "For many patients, the patient role, with its dependence on helping agencies, not only has become a way of life," Harris and Bergman state; "it has become their core and only identity" (1984, p. 30).

Even when these patients have been moved through treatment experiences that require progressively more responsibility—a strategy that presumably will enhance a positive identity—years of dysfunction may be too much to overcome without difficulty. Practitioners eager to help these persons may be quite discouraged when the persons show preferences for pathological definitions rather than socially accepted definitions of themselves. These clinicians may not appreciate the positive value that a patient identity can have (Harris & Bergman, 1984).

MacKinnon (1977) feels that the need for personal significance accounts for much postpsychotic depression. He speculates that significance and meaning can be nearly as important to human beings as food and sleep. As we have noted in Chapter 3 of this book, some patients may have considerable investment in their psychoses and feel real threats to their identity at the thought of giving them up. Two of MacKinnon's patients provided the following explanations:

I really missed my illness when I was free of it. I guess what I missed most was the sense of mystery. My visual hallucinations filled me with wonder and awe as well as scaring me more than any horror movie ever could have done. (p. 427)

My illness was a great ego builder. Just think, God thought I was so special he was punishing me like this. . . . It was quite a letdown to find that my "religious experience" was all a fraud and that people weren't really writing songs and magazine articles about me. (p. 427)

Identity is the nucleus of personality around which other ideas revolve—a person's concept of what he or she means, who he or she is, what he or she can do, and how he or she fits in the world. It includes likes, dislikes, roles, and personal characteristics. Erikson (1968), who focused much of his work on identity in adolescence and young adulthood, noted that present identity involves past identities, future aspirations, and contemporary cultural issues. If a person cannot bring together all the different facets of experience, he or she is said to suffer from "role diffusion." People who have had serious mental illnesses have had such a wide array of highly unusual experiences with their symptoms and treatment, not to mention stigma and rejection, that they face an enormous challenge to finding an acceptable identity.

Research instruments used to measure social adjustment assume that adjustment relates to the adoption of normative social roles (such as work and marriage), social contacts, and large social support networks. These goals are often unrealistic for men and women with serious psychiatric disturbances. The challenge for clinicians is to develop concepts of mental health appropriate to persons with mental illness.

OBSTACLES TO ACHIEVING AN ACCEPTABLE IDENTITY

Men and women with mental illnesses face many obstacles to developing an acceptable identity that others ordinarily do not face. Some of these barriers have their origins in the unique experiences of mental illness and their sequelae, and some in the ways that our society responds to them.

Community Acceptance of the Mentally Ill

It is generally accepted in developmental psychology that how we come to regard ourselves depends in part on the ways other regard us. If others regard us positively,we tend to see ourselves in an acceptable light, and a positive image becomes a part of our identity. As we have noted in Chapter 9, consumers frequently perceive themselves as being victims of rejection and discrimination, which they feel have their basis in stigma. Barbara Brundage (1983) explains:

> The stigma of mental illness was the hardest thing to overcome for me. I am embarrassed to admit how prejudiced I was. My attitude was, "It's ok for others, but it could never happen to me." It took me two years of intensive therapy, getting to know myself better, being fascinated, loving and hating it, to accept what I am. (p. 584)

An important concern of ours in this chapter is to note how social rejection affects the development of an acceptable identity. We know that the threat of being placed by others in a highly stigmatizing category such as "the mentally ill" leads to denial. Patients protect themselves against the degradation and depersonalization inherent in such a label by denying that they are mentally ill. Some patients restrict the label of "mentally ill" to fellow patients who they feel are clearly more disturbed than themselves (O'Mahoney, 1982).

Godschalx (1987) found that social rejection resulting from the stigma of mental illness produced significant existential dilemmas for patients, causing them to question their lives and to seek new meanings in their personal existences. Without successful resolution, severe demoralization and depression might occur. Godschalx, in a series of interviews found that patients used a variety of ego-protective explanations of their mental illnesses. For example, one interviewee said, "I do feel lots of people have nervous breakdowns. Apparently that's what happened to me" (p. 49). Another said, "I had a drug problem when I was 16. I come here . . . you guys are here to help people who don't go along with the social norm" (p. 49). A third said, "I think of myself as a normal person with some problems. I've come a long way to where I feel I'm not as bad as I used to be" (p. 55). According to O'Mahoney (1982), a limited degree of self-deception is normal within self-perception and serves important integrative functions within personality.

O'Mahoney studied the self-perceptions of 50 first-admission psychiatric patients as compared to their perceptions of the mentally ill and to the psychiatric staff's views of typical patients. The results showed that patients shared the staff's generally negative perceptions of the mentally ill, but that they did not see themselves in terms of this stereotype. It appears that people with mental illnesses themselves often tend to stigmatize and reject others who have these disorders.

These individuals may resist living with other mentally ill people, or may even reject the mental health system in its entirety (Hatfield, 1989).

Chapter 9 includes considerable discussion of efforts underway to reduce stigma through integrating people into the community, through providing opportunities for consumer-directed services, and through community education. There is some evidence that these efforts are on the right track and are paying off. According to Rabkin's (1984) summary of recent research regarding community attitudes toward the mentally ill, some changes are becoming apparent. Over the past 30 years, she reports, more than 100 studies have cumulatively demonstrated a current trend toward greater tolerance of mental patients. Open expressions of rejection of mental illness have declined over time. It is no longer socially acceptable to avoid and exclude persons labeled as mental patients simply on the grounds of their illness. However, people still tend to be apprehensive about having to deal with impaired mental patients and about their possible unpredictable and/or dangerous behavior.

Problems of social rejection may be more readily clarified and resolved if care is given to the use of terminology. It is social rejection that we are noting, and stigma may be only one of several explanations for the rejection. Several studies comparing public reactions to the label of "mental illness" and to the descriptions of disturbed behavior itself suggest that the behavior and not the label is what evokes the negative responses. Clausen's (1980) studies on labeling and attitudes toward the mentally ill leads him to conclude that it is deviant behavior, not the history of mental illness, that leads to labeling and/or rejection. This supports his contention that while mental illness is generally "devalued," the term "stigma" is misleading. The word "stigma" refers to reproach or disgrace that results from a label or from people's misconceptions of something. Because it is irrational, stigma can be difficult to counteract. In a case where social rejection is attributable to deviant behaviors that are offensive or intrusive to others, however, the change needs to occur within the individual, and rehabilitative techniques can be of help.

In cases where rejection is attributable to stigma, it is society that must change. Since this may not happen rapidly, we need to help people with mental illness develop as much imperviousness to the toxicity of stigma as we can. Difficult as it is to do, people can learn not to internalize these irrational attitudes. They can see this cruel behavior as someone else's problem and not something inherent in the disorder.

Social rejection can be a result of parochialism and ignorance. When people encounter a situation that is new to them, such as mental illness, they are uncertain how to behave and they become anxious. They may resent the person who they believe has made them feel so inadequate, so they may try to avoid contact with all mentally ill people. The answer in this case lies in helping others understand the behaviors of people with these disorders and offering them coping techniques that may be useful in certain situations.

Mental Illness Experiences and Their Sequelae

When we consider all that a person experiences in the course of a major mental illness, it is hard to understand how it is possible to integrate it all and develop a coherent self. As we have described earlier, during acute phases of such an illness patients suffer from alterations of their personal world, together with a disturbed sense of self involving loss of ego boundaries, confusion about identity, and a sense of being controlled by outside forces. Events are experienced as fragmentary, disjointed, and unpredictable. Intense feelings and hypersensitivity to others make interpersonal relationships highly tenuous, and loneliness is a constant companion.

The act of getting better poses additional threats to identity. Our society offers little help to those whose condition does not permit them to take on roles of school, work, marriage, and parenthood. The challenge for the mental health community is to find or create meaningful roles for those blocked from taking the more usual ones.

Some interesting recent research has investigated the structure of the self in schizophrenia. Gara, Rosenberg, and Mueller's (1989) study on the perceptions of self and others in schizophrenia found that those diagnosed with schizophrenia generally have poorly elaborated views of themselves relative to their views of other people. Their perceptions of others tend to be highly elaborated and stereotyped. In a more recent study using similar methodology, Robey, Cohen, and Gara (1989) produced similar findings about self structure, but did not confirm the same characteristics in the perception of others. Robey et al. noted that these studies could not confirm whether the self-structural deficits are primary deficits that precede or provide the conditions for other aspects of schizophrenic psychopathology, or are the results of more basic cognitive deficits.

FINDING MEANING IN LIFE

Godschalx (1987) based her phenomenological study of schizophrenic patients in the community on the existential question of meaning in human existence. Her assumption was that people with mental illnesses face a difficult predicament because they are usually unable to live what are considered "successful" lives, and therefore have particular difficulty in finding meaning in personal existence. Findings of her interview study of 30 patients living in the community indicated that the patients found a sense of meaning in a variety of less than traditional ways. An activity was meaningful if it offered one of the following two experiences: (1) a sense of accomplishment, or (2) a sense of usefulness. We use these two categories here to discuss the statements of personal meaning provided by the patients whose accounts we have examined.

A Sense of Accomplishment

Many patients express a sense of accomplishment in learning to accept and handle their illnesses. Nina, a patient quoted by Irvine (1985), feels that a person who has accomplished this can be a good example for others:

> You can show people who are going to have to deal with this illness most of their lives that it's OK, you can have a rewarding life, you can be functional, you can work a few hours a week, if not full time. You may not have all the "goodies," you may not be able to take off on a vacation whenever you want to, or buy a car, etc., but there are other things that make life rewarding. (p. 57)

> The other women in my age group are out there building empires, putting their energies into jobs and careers and buying condominiums and cars and doing things that people do. But something I have had to accept is that that is not going to be for me. And in accepting it, it takes away a lot of the remorse. (p. 56)

People with mental illnesses often express the feeling that their particular experiences equip them in very special ways to understand and help others. For example:

> Mental patients might be "crazy" but they are not "stupid." We believe that recovering psychiatric patients have a perspective from first-hand experience that is not available from anyone else, and that their expertise is useful and should be sought and respected. (Canadian Mental Health Association, 1985, p. iv)

Another patient quoted by Irvine (1985), Abigail, provides an elaboration of this concept:

It is part of the shamanic tradition — that it's wounded people who become the healers and that healing takes place reciprocally when people allow their wounds to be exposed and to accept help from each other. I think people who have had these awesome experiences and troubling experiences and have accepted the responsibility and challenge of integrating them are in a good position to give people motivation and hope. And it feels good to do that, which keeps you well. (p. 17)

Godschalx (1987) found that her subjects expressed accomplishment through working, "being the best," engaging in hobbies and sports, participating in therapy groups, and "getting well." "Doing something and doing it well" was the source of a sense of accomplishment and gave life meaning. Traditional employment was highly valued, as expressed by one of her interviewees:

. . . that was a fine job. I would drive a truck 10 hours and it wouldn't feel like it because I would be unloading trucks and ya know that's pretty fun to me. Having a pile of potatoes fall over, and having to pick them up again. *(laughter)* (p. 72)

Godschalx found that accomplishment was also experienced when people saw themselves as "being the best." In response to the questions "What do you enjoy in life?" one persons answered, "Knowing that I'm successful in the things I do. Like I can give an example such as an exercise group. I set the record for the amount of push-ups. To me that is really something" (p. 73).

Other meaningful roles were described in what are traditionally considered hobbies, such as crocheting and paint-by-number pictures. Godschalx says that considering these activities as "only hobbies" trivializes their importance in helping people experience accomplishment. Sports activities were another source of accomplishment, especially when a patient played an important role in winning a game. Other group activities might bring a sense of accomplishment, but as one person stated, they did not always do so:

Most of the groups are okay, but [the] cooking group is pretty shallow because there's not much potential in that, ya know. There's not a variety spectrum of things you can make, of things that you can really say that boy, that was what I made, ya know. (p. 73)

People whose capacities lie in the area of music and art may have a valuable resource upon which to draw. The creative and expressive abilities seem less affected by a major mental illness than do the cognitive abilities. One of us (Hatfield) knows three young men who seem to have found a sense of identity and accomplishment in the arts—two in the visual arts, and one in North Indian music. They work at their crafts on a daily basis and consider them their professions. Their families support them in these activities and feel that they have been crucial in their relatives' getting better.

Poetry is a constructive and meaningful outlet for some people. A recent publication titled *Cry of the Invisible,* edited by Susko (1991), illustrates the range of talent that resides in people with serious mental illnesses.

A Sense of Being Useful

Experiencing usefulness, or being needed, gave life meaning for some of Godschalx's (1987) subjects. Caring for parents or other family members was a frequently mentioned role, that was not anticipated by the researcher. Two of her examples, the first one showing the importance of a caring role and the second the sense of uselessness without that role, follow:

> I take care of my mom. She needs me and I've only got one mom. It makes me feel useful cause it helps my mom, ya know. (p. 74)

> On Social Security the first couple of months I thought I would go nuts. I felt like I wasn't needed in the world, ya know. Just existing one day to the next, I had to do something, make my life worth something, ya know. (p. 74)

Work is what gives meaning and a sense of identity to most people in our society, and this is equally true of those with serious mental illnesses. Godschalx's subjects associated going to work with normality. As one woman said:

> Normal is the person that gets ups and goes to work in the morning and sometimes has breakfast and sometimes doesn't and they have their loves, they have their hates. They have their jobs and sometimes it is difficult and sometimes it is easy and most of the time it gets pretty routine. They do the same thing over and over again and they don't have to worry too much. They just live their lives. (p. 82)

But most studies show that few mentally ill people actually have competitive employment. Only two people in the Canadian Mental Health

Association (1985) study were engaged in full-time, full-paying employment. Of all community needs, this was most often mentioned. A middle-aged woman in this study said:

> Yes, I had to work full time. I always worked. It's my life. In order for me to get back to normal living, I had to get back to an eight-thirty to five day. There was no way I could live a normal life and not get up in the morning to go to work. (p. 21)

The struggle for this group to find work was often overwhelming. They attributed most of their problems in this regard to stigma. They struggled with the issue of lying or telling the truth about their psychiatric histories, and frequently took themselves out of the job market to avoid the anxiety over this deception. People felt that they were being pushed by others to go out and find a job, yet the reality was often a profoundly negative experience. "I tried to get jobs, I tried, I tried, I got laid off," one person said; another said simply, "The jobs are not there" (Canadian Mental Health Association, 1985, p. 23).

Some people with mental illnesses capitalize on their personal knowledge of mental illness to work with others with similar problems. Increasingly we hear about drop-in centers being organized by recovering patients. Daniel Link (Chapter 14, this volume) wrote a grant application and received funding for the Self-Help Center, a social center in St. Louis, Missouri, which employs only recovering patients.

Mental health consumers with chronic mental illnesses are being trained for employment as case management aides in a psychiatric rehabilitation project in Denver. In initiating the project, the Colorado Division of Mental Health assumed that people with lengthy experiences as consumers of services in the mental health and social services systems had some useful experience and might be able to establish rapport more quickly with other consumers. At a 2-year follow-up of the program, 17 of the original 25 trainees for the program were employed as case management aides (Sherman & Porter, 1991).

According to the authors of this report, the success of the project was reflected in changed attitudes of staff and consumers in the system. Those in the professional mental health community were forced to change their pessimistic predictions about the potential abilities of clients for this kind of work, and other training projects are being developed. Writing in a local newsletter for patients and families, one case management aide said:

> . . . work can help reduce the stigma of mental illness by proving to other clients, to providers, and to the general public that, with the right type and amount of support, persons who have experienced

severe mental illness can become productive, contributing members
of their communities. (quoted in Sherman & Porter, 1991, p. 498)

In a book entitled *Wounded Healers,* Rippere and Williams (1985)
bring together stories written by people who not only have suffered
from severe depression but are also professionals in the mental health
service system. Included are psychiatrists, psychologists, psychiatric
nurses, social workers, and occupational therapists. Some were already
in the system at the time of their depressive episode. For others, it was
the crucial determinant in their choice of profession.

The autobiographical accounts in *Wounded Healers* demonstrate
the gap between the complex and changing experiential sides of depression and the neat diagnostic categories that occur in professional literature. One reaction to this dilemma is to transcend one's own experience
of being poorly understood by providing a service that is empathic and
compassionate. Rippere and Williams draw on the work of Bennett
(1979) to explain the title of their book, as well as the unique contri-
bution that can be made by people with depressive conditions or other
major mental illnesses.

Bennett (1979) says that in many cultures the healer will also be
a sufferer. This is true in societies where there are shamans, as noted
above by Irvine's (1985) informant Abigail. These people are thought
to have a mixture of priestly and healing powers, but they also pos-
sess some defect, which in the Western world might be an illness or
disability of some kind. Rippere and Williams (1985) find these traditional beliefs regarding the "wounded healer" relevant to the issue of
transmuting the stigma of mental illness into a potentially positive asset.

Paulson (1991) directs a unique program in Cincinnati, Ohio,
called the Specialized Mental Health Training Program. The aim is
to empower consumers and family members by recruiting them into
the program, which is designed to prepare people in social work to
work with the seriously mentally ill and their families. Basic to the
program is the assumption that the consumers' and family members'
experiences should be viewed as assets that should be preserved and
utilized to enhance the learning of professional colleagues and bring
about positive changes in the service system. At the same time, the
consumers and their relatives develop a sense of competence, self-
esteem, and acceptable identity.

SUMMARY AND IMPLICATIONS

This chapter has focused on the process by which recovering patients
develop an acceptable identity and meaningful goals in their lives. This

is an existential task that faces all individuals, but it is an especially daunting task for people who face an array of problems inherent in having a mental illness. Young chronic patients strive for independence, satisfying relationships, a sense of identity, and a realistic vocational choice. Lacking the ability to withstand stress and intimacy, they struggle and fail repeatedly; the results are often anxiety, depression, psychotic episodes, and apathy (Lamb, 1982). Lamb advises that we work with younger patients while they are still motivated to do something and support realistic goals. Once these people get older and have experienced repeated failures, they may be all too willing to settle for life without goals and a low level of functioning.

Engagement, Lamb says, is the therapeutic answer to meaninglessness. He quotes the existential psychotherapist I. D. Yalom on ways of overcoming meaninglessness:

> To find a home, to care about other individuals, about ideas or projects, to search, to create, to build—these, and all other forms of engagement, are twice rewarding: they are intrinsically enriching, and they alleviate the dysphoria that stems from being bombarded with the unassembled brute data in existence. (Lamb, 1982, p. 468)

But Jones (1975) has questioned whether we know enough to help people develop a life style and activities that will lead to the goals outlined by Yalom and will provide a sense of accomplishment and self-fulfillment. He feels that a new philosophy of care is needed, in which we help patients find their hidden potential and develop a therapeutic culture of their own.

Undoubtedly, we still have a long way to go before we can truly say that we understand the internal struggles of people with mental disorders for a meaningful existence and an acceptable identity. Even when we do begin to understand, we face an enormous challenge to our imagination and creativity to respond in helpful ways. There is some evidence in the current literature, however, that attempts at such responses are underway.

CHAPTER THIRTEEN

Learning to Manage
the Illness
and Avoid Relapse

At this point in psychiatric history, professionals are beginning to recognize the strengths and inner resources of patients themselves in managing their own illnesses. Involved are a range of endeavors: self-education about the illnesses; self-monitoring to avoid decompensation; compliance with prescribed medication regimens and rejection of self-medication through substance abuse; participation in activities for personal growth and mutual support; attempts to recapture the lost developmental stages of learning through education or job training; and, above all, attitudinal change from denial to acceptance of the illness. The last of these includes both a recognition of personal limitations and an ability to find creative alternatives to transcend them. Implicit in illness management is the element of hope—the expectation that despite the illness, a patient, like other human beings, can attain a reasonably satisfying quality of life.

Before going into the actual techniques that patients have developed for themselves and have disclosed through research to others, we must begin with the basic groundwork of illness management: that is, the meaning and salience of the illness to each patient, and the conditions under which patients wish to control symptoms and avoid relapse.

PSYCHODYNAMIC ISSUES
IN ILLNESS MANAGEMENT

Illness management is first of all contingent on patients' acknowledgment that they have a disability—that they are not functioning as well as they should be. The modes of illness management are further determined by patients' motivation for change. This means an acceptance of the need to adapt their own ways of perceiving reality in the service of illness control. It also includes patients' willingness to develop their own monitoring strategies and to utilize techniques taught by others (e.g., Liberman et al., 1986). In Chapter 2, we have discussed a number of questions regarding the parameters of patients' volition and control over internal events. There is continuing debate over the gap between capability and motivation to use available degrees of control to avoid decompensation. The major issue underlying this gap is the psychodynamic meaning of the illness to the patient.

When we speak of the psychodynamic meaning of the illness in relation to motivation, it is clear that for many patients there is an ongoing, overarching struggle between recognizing and acknowledging their limitations, and their desire to be perceived and to function as normal members of society. This involves tensions between two needs: dependency on others for survival, and maintenance of ego integrity by affirming the ability to function independently. A patient who has not been able to graduate from high school or obtain a general education diploma because of attentional and cognitive deficits may announce intentions of becoming a lawyer or engineer—goals that are deterrents to preparing for the less demanding but lower-level jobs he or she may be able to learn in vocational training or transitional employment. Here, the symptom of grandiosity is a maladaptive coping strategy in illness management. Masking a fear of being tested, the grandiosity also protects against loss of dependency status.

The system attempts to deal with these dependency issues in many ways. In supportive psychotherapy, the aim is to curtail dependency needs by building self-esteem and indicating directions in which the client may become more autonomous. In rehabilitation, the aim is to reinforce existing competencies and develop actual skills—social, interpersonal, and occupational—that will enable the person to function more independently. All interventions try to remove the self-stigmatization that typically interferes with the person's acknowledgment that he or she has some deficits requiring remediation or change.

The rise of patients' organizations has been one way in which people have begun to acknowledge their status as present or former consumers of mental health services. Some defiantly identify themselves as mental patients, but continue to deny the condition that gave rise to this status. Many more, however, are acknowledging that they have an illness that requires management, and are educating themselves as much as possible about their diagnosis and treatment.

SELF-EDUCATION
AND EDUCATING OTHERS

The system is finally becoming aware of the need to educate patients about their symptoms and to teach coping skills and enhance existing competencies. Psychoeducational groups for patients are increasingly being used; patients in these groups learn symptom recognition and control, as well as self-behavior management strategies (Corrigan, Davies-Farmer, & Lome, 1988; Liberman, 1987; Liberman et al., 1986). Corrigan, Liberman, and Engel (1990) describe a program to move persons with schizophrenia from noncompliance to collaboration. They teach patients and families about the biomedical nature of mental illness and its relation to stress; identify and use reinforcers; and apply cognitive restructuring techniques to elicit attitude change and remotivation. Patients are specifically taught about medications—self-administration, identifying side effects, negotiating medication issues with health service providers, and symptom management. Patients learn to identify warning signs of relapse, to manage warning signs, to recognize and cope with persistent symptoms, and to avoid alcohol and street drugs.

Unfortunately, these programs are available only in limited locations, and many persons who might benefit do not have access to systematic patient education. Some people, however, are highly motivated to study, and will spend many hours and days in libraries researching their own syndromes and even arriving at their own diagnoses. In a class conducted by one of us (Lefley) with second-year psychiatric residents, a former patient with a diagnosis of schizophrenia described in detail his reactions to specific neuroleptics and the mode in which he believed they affected his own dopamine system—and was knowledgeable enough to elicit respectful questions from the physicians being educated.

Another former patient who has received multiple diagnoses described "reading everything in sight" in order to arrive at a self-diagnosis that made sense to her. Furthermore, she charted her symptoms and responses to various medications in order to make informed treatment decisions. At a meeting on managed care at the National Conference on Mental Health Statistics, she presented a paper describing two major coping responses that enabled her to deal with her illness, a major affective disorder (Loder, 1991). One was to organize a support group by soliciting the local mental health association for a meeting room and recruiting other patients through newspaper ads— measures that ultimately led to a number of area support groups and a consumer advocacy movement. The other coping strategy was to set up her own system of managed care by maintaining a daily personal journal. In her presentation, Loder (1991) described how she used her own data system to monitor symptom change and medication response. She described "strange episodes where sounds became distant, a sensation of dizziness, extreme anxiety, and the world being off-kilter came over me" (p. 5). These episodes also included involuntary body movements. But "I didn't talk about that because I was already considered 'mentally ill' . . . After studying my journals, there was an obvious relation between the frequency, duration, and intensity of these experiences and the dosage of a particular medication I was taking" (p. 5). These episodes were later diagnosed as temporal lobe seizures, and with her doctor's agreement she gradually reduced her medications. Loder emphasizes a need for the system to look beyond people's limitations and "to provide people the opportunities we all deserve—to grow, change, take control of our lives, and heal" (1991, p. 6).

Still other people have learned how to take control of their lives by disclosing their needs to others and shaping a desired mode of interaction. A former patient has described how she educated others to listen and take her seriously:

> There was a general attitude that because I was an ex-psychiatric inmate, I couldn't possibly have any good ideas or anything of value to say. I've fought to make myself heard, and I do feel now that people listen to me, and that they pay attention to what I'm saying. I had to say to people at times, "I don't want to be treated like an inmate. I want to be treated as if what I say is of some value, and is as valid as anything anyone else says." (quoted in Campbell, 1989b, p. 33)

SELF-MONITORING AND SYMPTOM MANAGEMENT

In the process of studying the experiences of schizophrenia, Strauss (1989b) recollects a patient's demanding, "Why don't you ever ask what I do to help myself?" He points out that "what she and others suggest is that the person as an active agent interacts with mental disorder in a crucial way that influences the course of that disorder" (1989b, p. 182). In the preceding section we have discussed a type of systematic self-monitoring through charting symptoms and responses to medications. Although few patients follow such a comprehensive procedure, there is evidence that many people with major mental illnesses are aware of their mental and emotional states, and try to prevent exacerbation of their symptoms.

Leete (1989), for example, describes her hypervigilance to repetitive noises or other multiple environmental stimuli, and her efforts to reduce distraction in order to avoid excessive nervousness and irritability. She reports forcing herself to attempt some kind of eye contact in order to ease social situations, and, conversely, temporarily withdrawing to another room when social interaction becomes too overwhelming. To counteract paranoid fears of being surprised, she chooses a seat where she can face the door and have her back to the wall, and provides herself with reality checks by asking other people whom they are calling or where they are going. She makes an effort not to talk to her voices in the presence of others, actively seeks social support, and deals with impaired concentration by writing down important information. Leete's personal warning signs of decompensation include

> fatigue or decreased sleep; difficulty with concentration and memory; increased paranoia, delusions, and hallucinations; tenseness and irritability; agitation; and being more easily overwhelmed by my surroundings. Coping mechanisms may include withdrawing and being alone for awhile; obtaining support from a friend; socializing or otherwise distracting myself from stressors; organizing my thoughts through lists; problem-solving around specific issues; or temporarily increasing my medication. (1989, pp. 199–200)

Medication Compliance and Monitoring

Unlike Leete, many patients not only are unwilling to increase medications, but are likely to decrease or eliminate them as soon as they begin to feel better. Many studies indicate that patient compliance with treatment prescriptions is extremely poor. Corrigan et al. (1990) cite the following barriers to patient collaboration: side effects; a complex treatment regimen and long-term treatment; patient characteristics, such as cognitive disorganization, ignorance about the illness, a fatalistic attitude, and/or possible secondary gain from psychosis; family characteristics, such as ignorance about the benefits of treatment, unrealistic expectations, and/or an indifferent attitude; clinician characteristics, such as an aversive interpersonal style, a belief that the patient has a poor prognosis, and/or disregard for the patient's dissatisfaction with treatment; and treatment delivery system characteristics, such as an aversive clinic setting, long waits at the clinic, and/or lack of coordination of services.

Special medication management skills can be taught to patients with serious mental illness, to enable them to monitor effects of antipsychotic drugs on a daily basis and to report side effects or early warning signs of relapse (Eckman, Liberman, & Phipps, 1990). Corrigan et al. (1990) also spell out ways in which family and clinician characteristics can be changed, and barriers in the clinician–patient relationship can be corrected. Above all, by endowing patients with information, skills, and instructions, mental health professionals will be able to empower the patients to take control of their own treatment. Patients become instructors of their therapists on how best to do this, through individual clinical interactions and through the research process.

Recognizing Prodromal Cues and Preventing Decompensation

To study the symptoms preceding psychotic episodes, Herz (1984) conducted interviews with one group of family members and two groups of schizophrenic patients—one whose psychotic episodes had just occurred, and one whose episodes had occurred 6 months earlier. In both groups, approximately 70% of the patients answered "yes" to the question "Could you tell that there were any changes in your thoughts, feelings, or behaviors that might have led you to believe that you were becoming sick and might have to go to the hospital?" Among family members, 93% responded that they could notice changes in the patients.

> Generally, the patients and family members most frequently reported nonpsychotic symptoms, or the type of dysphoria that nonpsychotic individuals experience under stress, such as feeling tense and nervous, eating less, having trouble concentrating, having trouble sleeping, feeling depressed, and seeing friends less. The nonpsychotic symptom reported by most patients in both groups was becoming tense and nervous, and the psychotic symptom most frequently reported was a feeling of being laughed at or talked about. (Herz, 1984, p. 345)

The purpose of this study was to develop a strategy of early therapeutic intervention to recognize prodromal cues and avert full-blown psychosis. However, only half of the individual patients noted a similar pattern of prodromal symptoms each time they relapsed; the other half reported that the prodromal cues varied. One of the reasons was that many of the symptoms, such as tension and nervousness, feeling sad, and worrying, were also present during periods of wellness.

The overreaching factor in decompensation appears to be stress. In earlier research, Herz and Melville (1980) reported that approximately 33% of the patients and their relatives were able to relate relapse to a stressful life event, such as job loss or marital problems. In the later research, patients questioned weeks or months after a relapse were generally not able to identify a specific event leading to symptom recurrence: "However, almost all patients interviewed during a prodromal phase were able to identify a specific event as a precipitant" (Herz, 1984, p. 347). A similar pattern was observed in international research conducted by the World Health Organization, in which subjects from many cultures reported specific stressful life events in the 3 weeks preceding onset of an acute schizophrenic episode (Day et al., 1987). Herz (1984) reported that prodromal phases usually lasted more than a week. Therefore, relapse was not abrupt and might have been averted through appropriate crisis interventions.

The Person–Disorder Interaction

How motivated are individual patients to share information on their prodromal states and enlist the help of professionals in preventing a psychotic episode? Strauss (1989b) has pointed out that the subjective experiences of mental illness—the modes in which the individual interacts with the disorder—are critically related to the interpretation and management of symptoms. "These person–disorder interactions involve the person as a goal-directed being; the patient's feelings, interpretations, and actions influencing phases of disorder and improvement; and the existence of regulatory mechanisms that guide the evolution of these phases" (p. 182). Patients' feelings about the disorder, and their perception of the current situation, influence the subsequent management and evolution of the illness. For example, cycles of remission and reactivation of symptoms—an agonizing history of raised and dashed hopes—will affect subsequent efforts to improve symptoms or control decompensation. An experience of improvement followed by relapse has an "immense impact on active role and subsequent experience. . . . Improvement for such a patient can acquire a meaning—'look out, you're just going to get your hopes up and then fall apart again' " (Strauss, 1989b, p. 183)

Dealing with Voices

Other patients, however, may work out means of living with their symptoms, so that they do not interfere with productivity or impair the person's quality of life. Strauss (1989b) and others (Benjamin, 1989) note that hearing voices may be frightening, but that the voices may also have companionship and advice-giving functions. They may even help the patient develop negotiating skills. Strauss describes a case in which the patient at first felt the voices were hostile and inimical to his efforts to get ahead in life. Increasingly finding it hard to ignore or even capitulate to the voices, he began to negotiate and come to some *modus vivendi* with them. Strauss noted that

> this young man, still being seen in followup interviews, already finds this negotiation seems to allow him to progress further with his ambitions than has been possible previously. He is hopeful . . . that this approach may help him to succeed where before he had met only with increased intensity of his voices and with failure, frustration, and relapse. (1989b, p. 183)

Benjamin (1989), however, feels that voices serve an interactional function missing in the social environment, and in contrast to Strauss, maintains that "the more adaptive the relationship with the hallucination, the more intractable and chronic the illness" (p. 308).

The Role of Insight

How important is insight in illness management? Greenfield et al. (1989) conducted a series of interviews with patients recovering from acute psychotic disorders and found that "patients presented an amazingly broad range of views about their psychoses" (p. 247). With respect to symptomatology, "our subjects' reports ranged over a continuum from massive denial of symptoms to detailed discussion and clear description of them" (p. 247). More than half (52%) either denied or trivialized their symptoms, or else presented "a complex mixture of acknowledgement and denial " (p. 247). Only 48% gave a reasonably detailed discussion of their symptoms. Moreover, "acknowledgement and description of psychotic symptoms did not necessarily lead patients to identify themselves as suffering from an illness" (p. 248). In fact, 64% of the patients who were able to give detailed symptom descriptions denied the existence of psychiatric illness. "A majority of patients . . . regarded the experience as perhaps reflecting a considerable problem but still as an isolated and unique event in their lives" (p. 248). Yet all dreaded relapse, and the thought of recurrent psychosis generated intense anxiety.

Illness management appears to be related to the developmental course of the disorder, the person's evaluation of symptoms, and the effectiveness of various methods used to control them. Timing appears to be important, but it is hard to determine patterns in the interaction of the course of illness, internal motivation, external events, and the salience or adverse loading of particular symptoms. Strauss (1989b) notes:

> In a series of interviews with persons who had improved after 10 years or more of severe mental disorder, several suggested that a key point for them was a change in attitude. . . . Somehow, after an extended period, they found themselves wanting not just to live with their illness but to have a life along with it or in spite of it. Some stated that they came to accept their disorders. But this was not the kind of giving-up acceptance or resignation that often seems generated by the attempts some professionals make at helpful teaching (e.g., "You have an illness like diabetes and will have it all your life. You'll need to stay on medication and there are certain things you'll never be able to do.") The acceptance described by these subjects was one that involved hope for a better life and the resolve to work for it. In several instances, subjects noted that symptoms — even delusions or hallucinations — then started to become less dominating and often faded considerably. (p. 184)

Strauss also designates a number of "regulatory mechanisms," such as modes of response to auditory hallucinations, that help individuals handle their symptoms and thus adjust to the illness. He suggests that so-called "negative symptoms" may have a regulatory function: "Apathy, withdrawal, and muteness may reflect a self-protective mechanism that the person with severe mental disorder uses to avoid the numerous discouragements and psychological assaults inflicted by the disorder, by society, and even by oneself" (1989b, p. 184). As we will see, they may also be modes of protecting oneself from an over-stimulating environment.

INTERACTION OF BIOLOGICAL NEEDS AND ILLNESS MANAGEMENT STRATEGIES

Program staff members should be particularly aware of certain illness management strategies that may appear to be maladaptive because they run counter to programmatic planning in most mental health systems. There is a tension here between programmatic demands oriented toward optimal functioning or normality, and patients' setting their own limits on the amount of normality they are able to manage. Within patients themselves, there is a tension between meeting their own expressed desires and goals — goals that are consonant with cultural expectations of adults in our society — and the biologically based needs imposed by their illness.

There is an increasing and generally salutary press toward normalization of persons with mental illnesses. The move toward supported housing, for example, is an effort to place deinstitutionalized patients in their own apartments in scattered sites, instead of in group homes or "mental health ghettos" with other patients. One of the concerns about this is the reinforcement of patients' tendencies toward social isolation. If they are removed from the peer supports and friendships of people with whom they have lived for a long time, will this not add to decompensation? Researchers have noted that in the histories of persons with schizophrenia, many patients had already manifested a withdrawal from social contact prior to their first episode. Taken as a prodromal symptom, this behavior may instead have been an effort to protect against the stress of interpersonal interactions. Spring (1981) notes that although social isolation may seem unpleasant to a neutral observer, "To a preschizophrenic who possibly harbors different preconceptions about the value of social isolation, they may seem well worth the cost" (p. 30). Spring claims that social isolation has often represented goal-oriented behavior—a coping strategy to avert interpersonal stress. In these cases isolation preceded rather than averted psychosis, however. It is evident that the disruption of social supports and the ease of decompensation permitted by an isolated life make this behavior highly maladaptive.

Nevertheless, persons with a major mental illness like schizophrenia may indeed manifest their inability to tolerate high levels of environmental stimulation or expectation in the treatment environment by withdrawing to smoke or walk around. Some may refuse to get up in the morning or to participate in program activities because they find this too demanding. It is often difficult for staff members to judge whether these behaviors reflect laziness, defiance, or other ways in which patients try to wrest control over their lives from other people, or whether they actually reflect an adaptive response to a biological need to control hyperarousal. This is one of the reasons why it is so important for staff members to know their patients and to gear expectations to each individual in their treatment planning. Too often, program evaluation depends on fulfillment of global requirements for quantified behavioral goals, rather than on individuals' movement in relation to their baseline behaviors and to realistic personal goals.

PATIENTS' ORGANIZATIONS IN ILLNESS MANAGEMENT

Patients' organizations are one of the most fruitful ways of offering meaning to a life too often seen as meaningless by a patient and others.

Joining with other patients, or working on behalf of other patients, has become what is surely one of the most adaptive means of illness management. Education of self and others, including public education; advocacy and political action; jobs in communication and information dissemination; roles in mental health service delivery; peer support and socialization; and avenues of self-fulfillment—all of these offer wonderfully adaptive ways of dealing with illness formerly viewed as demoralizing and demeaning.

Some problems with patients' movements, however, may lead to maladaptive illness management. One is the still unresolved issue of acknowledging mental illness. We have previously spoken of divisions in the consumer movement, which essentially involve two conflicting views. One is that "mental illness" is an unclear and perhaps spurious concept—that behaviors so labeled are largely products of the psychiatric establishment and of treatment of patients in the mental health system. This is a Szaszian view, with a major adaptive function of fueling anger in persons who are intact enough to use it. The adaptive aspects of anger enable formerly demoralized persons to subscribe to a cause that infuses purpose into their lives. The maladaptive aspects, of course, range from denial to rejection of treatment for themselves and for others who may desperately need it.

The other view is that mental illnesses are indeed valid—that DSM entities are properly described and differentiated—but that patients who have these illnesses can manage them through proper medication and support systems, particularly through developing their own management techniques. These latter individuals still function politically, but they act to improve rather than to tear down the service delivery system. Thus one type of person manages the illness through denial and anger; the other does so through acceptance, self-monitoring, and self-improvement.

An increasingly evident problem is that of overwork on the part of members of the consumer leadership. The overwhelming tasks involved in building organizations, welding together factions, developing constituencies, and maintaining balanced budgets are difficult and demanding even for the most high-functioning individuals. Consumer-operated services impose further demands and frustrations, well known to the majority of staff members in most service delivery systems. Some persons in leadership roles will have illness-related problems that may include attentional deficits, sensitivity to stimulus arousal, or just plain tiredness. The retarding effects or extrapyramidal symptoms of specific psychotropic medications will add to difficulties in fulfilling the demanding organizational tasks. It may be predicted that some persons with a history of psychiatric illness, no matter how strong and talented, may be unable to deal with these combined stressors. Indeed, in some cases, overworked leaders have decompensated and required rehospitalization. Strauss's (1989b) caution—that a relapse may convey such a discouraging message that it interferes with subsequent recovery—must be taken into account. The preparation of talented persons for consumer leadership roles should include the message that relapses may very well occur, but that no connotation of failure is attached to them and that periods of hospitalization need not interfere with subsequent performance roles.

The most salutary form of illness management is found among persons who are well educated about their conditions, and who control their own lives through self-monitoring of symptoms and treatment response. Acceptance of the illness brings optimal control, because it permits clients to develop their own preventative schemas for avoiding the loss of autonomy. At a 1990 Consumer Roundtable on Alternatives to Involuntary Treatment, sponsored by the Community Support Program of the National Institute of Mental Health (Blanch, 1990), consumers suggested a number of strategies that would make involuntary intervention less likely or necessary. These included behavioral contracts, living wills, crisis cards, and durable power of attorney. All of these are proactive mechanisms that permit psychiatric patients to make competent decisions about their own future treatment, to take effect only if they lose the capacity for rational decision. "Involuntary" treatment is thus precluded by the specific directions of potential patients about what they want other people to be allowed (or not allowed) to do to them in the event of decompensation.

In describing the global consumer movement, we have previously noted the differentiation between advocacy and self-help or mutual support groups. In most support groups the members acknowledge the validity of their illnesses and learn how to cope with them. One former patient attributes her ability to cope with schizophrenia to specific "self-help tools" learned as a member of Recovery, Inc. These include "the tool of humor to laugh over situations that formerly made me tense" (McKenzie, 1982, p. 19). They also include a kind of self–other differentiation by deliberately shifting from thinking about the self to thinking about the needs of others and putting herself in the other person's situation. One of the major coping skills she learned was how to deal with paranoid ideation or delusional thoughts about other people:

> I take the secure thought if I start to worry about what strangers think of me that . . . nine times out of ten, people have more important things to think about than me. I drop the exaggerated sense

of my importance in other people's lives and my tenseness goes.
(McKenzie, 1982, p. 19)

HOW THE SYSTEM CAN
HELP PATIENTS HELP THEMSELVES

Promotion of Creative Expression

For psychiatrically disabled persons, one of the most difficult aspects
of illness management is reconciling their known talents and skills with
a narrow window of occupational opportunities. Often, the only jobs
available are physically demanding and intellectually stultifying. The
clinician is always in a bind regarding the actual potential of an individual who may indeed be too talented and intelligent for the entry-
level jobs available in most vocational training programs. These jobs
may be viewed as demeaning and as threatening to the ego integrity
of a person who has not forgotten past academic triumphs and skills.
Some clients may be able to turn their talents to writing, painting, or
other artistic pursuits. These are proactive attempts to overcome the
boundaries imposed by illness. Although a major psychotic disorder
may preclude competitive employment in occupations that a client
knows are consonant with his or her past skills, creative expression
is an excellent mode of illness management. It provides an outlet for
the client's skills and an educational and artistic experience for the
audience toward whom the works are targeted.

There is a clear role for clinicians and consumer advocates in
promoting the artistic expressions of persons with serious mental illness. Many of the citations in this book are from clients' writings published in compilations by the National Alliance for the Mentally Ill
and in *Schizophrenia Bulletin*. Clients' writings have also been com-
piled by consumer groups themselves, such as the client-directed California Well-Being Project, which has provided both research findings
(Campbell, 1989a) and an anthology of art, poetry, prose, and photography (Campbell, 1989b).

On the artistic front, National Art Exhibitions by the Mentally
Ill, Inc., is a national exhibit of paintings and sculptures of clients of
state hospitals, community mental health centers, and other programs
throughout the United States serving persons with severe and persistent mental illnesses. Initiated by a group of community mental health
workers in Miami, Florida, the juried exhibit is selected from submis-
sions by a panel of art experts. Patients price their own works and

receive the full amount when they are sold. In 5 years of exhibitions, almost all works have been sold. This enterprise familiarizes the public with the artistic talents and productivity of persons, many of them currently in institutions, who are clearly identified as mentally ill. It also provides a source of income to patients, and allows them to enhance their talents and self-esteem in art competitions viewed by large numbers of the community. The destigmatization of the process is confirmed by the substantial number of patients (the majority of exhibitors) who wish their names to be publicized in connection with their art.

It should be strongly cautioned that literary or artistic productive expression of talent is very different from art as diagnostic or psychodynamic material. The first connotes creativity within a normalizing role, the other the interpretive contents of psychopathology. An artist/patient has stated:

> In all the time that I was in treatment programs and in hospitals I would never have tried to draw a picture or paint. No matter what kind of picture you draw in a hospital, a therapist will pick it up and try to apply some sort of secret meaning to it. Whereas now, a few times I have noticed myself picking up a blank piece of paper and sketching. It's that freedom, when I don't feel I'm being judged, that lets me do it. (quoted in Campbell, 1989b, p. 115)

Supported University Education

In the examples given above, the system has provided mechanisms for clients to function creatively within the parameters of their status as persons with mental illnesses. In these endeavors, patients use their expertise to educate others about the experiences, dilemmas, and inner thoughts of persons with psychiatric disabilities. Their expertise provides a coping mechanism for self-expression, self-healing, and educating the world about mental illness.

The system also provides other avenues for personal growth that enable persons with mental illnesses to continue their education and to enhance their employment potential. A model supported education program is offered by Boston University's Center for Psychiatric Rehabilitation. The center recently reported on a study of 52 young adults with severe psychiatric disabilities who voluntarily applied for and participated in a four-semester program. The curriculum consisted of four instructional sections related to career development: profiling vocational potential, researching occupational alternatives, career planning, and mobilizing personal skills and competencies. Thirty-five of the subjects completed the program, and after the intervention 42% of the students were competitively employed or enrolled in an educational program, compared with 19% before the intervention. There was also a significant decrease in hospitalizations, as well as a significant increase in self-esteem (Unger, Anthony, Sciarappa, & Rogers, 1991).

SUMMARY AND CONCLUSIONS

It is important for mental health professionals to realize that management of psychiatric illnesses ultimately depends on the patients themselves. This chapter has indicated how some persons with major illnesses develop and apply their own strategies for illness management and prevention of decompensation. Patients develop methods for educating themselves about their illnesses. They read, study, maintain journals to observe their own reactions, and educate others in how to treat them so they can maintain ego integrity and self-esteem. They describe their self-monitoring strategies to handle paranoid ideation, techniques to screen out environmental stimuli that interfere with information processing, and ways of accommodating to "voices" or other persistent hallucinatory material. They learn to accept medications, to monitor their responses to them, to assess side effects, and to share this information with professionals.

Patients are able to recognize prodromal cues of decompensation and to deal with them directly (e.g., through avoiding fatigue or eliminating potential stressors) or indicating (through soliciting professional aid). Illness management appears to be related to the developmental course of the disorder, the person's evaluation of symptoms, and the perceived effectiveness of the various methods used to control or transcend the symptoms. Improvement seems to be related to motivation for change rather than to insight. Patients who improve do more than accept their limitations: They resolve to live with their illness but to work for a better quality of life.

In this chapter we have talked about the interaction of biological needs and illness management strategies. "Negative symptoms" such as withdrawal may sometimes serve a self-protective function. It is important for professionals to realize that there is often a tension between programmatic demands and the amount of stimulation that a particular patient can tolerate. Illness management sometimes consists of patients setting their own limits on the environmental demands they are able to manage. Staff members must learn to differentiate between laziness, resistance, or even hostile defiance, and a biological need to control hyperarousal.

CHAPTER FOURTEEN

Life on the Ledge:
My Recovery from a
Major Mental Illness
A Consumer's Personal Recollection

DANIEL LINK, M.S.W.

On May 26, 1985, I walked out the front door of my home, leaving my wife and two stepsons (aged 1 and 6) behind. Down the long gravel driveway I walked. I approached the mailbox gingerly, knowing what it might contain. And there it was, my report card for my first semester at the University of Missouri–St. Louis. I had returned to school as a junior social work student and had taken, out of sequence, five required courses. The grade column contained only A's. Despite what I had achieved over the past 1½ years, I felt that this was when my recovery from schizophrenia was complete.

The contrast to December 1974 could not have been more striking. At that time, I was 22 years old and was in the psychiatric unit of Barnes Hospital, St. Louis, Missouri. Over the next 2 months, I would have 12 shock treatments and would experience, for the first time, the effects of antipsychotic medication. At that point in time, I believed that the U.S. government was drugging the food of the populace; that the government was tapping my phone, my house, and my television; that there were two distinct classes of Americans—those involved in the conspiracy to drug and silence the general population, and the majority of Americans, whom I believed the conspirators were controlling; and that with the conflict of Vietnam and the influx of drugs into our society, narcotics were illegal because they counteracted the drugs that "they" were putting into our food and drink. It would be many years before I broke out of this delusional world view.

My delusional thought system had actually begun in February 1973, and it would last until November 1983. At no time during these 10 years did I break through this delusional world view as outlined above. During this time period, I spent approximately 450 days as an inpatient in public and private psychiatric hospitals. I was labeled as a dangerous and noncompliant patient. Prolixin Decanoate was developed during this period and biweekly injections helped to keep me out of trouble, but not completely. I was arrested at least five times— including an arrest for arson, committed for what I thought at the time was a good reason. All actions leading to arrests were related to my belief system. In fact, I believed that I was a patriot for challenging the government's control of the population. I regularly drank rainwater and urine, believing that all other commercially prepared drinks (and even the water from the faucet) were drugged. I ate feces more than once for the same reason. I abused illicit drugs.

Looking back now, I can present a pretty convincing argument that my belief system was insane, not my actions. My actions were consistent with the world that I believed I lived in. These 10 years of illness comprised my 20s—a time during which most adults marry and begin families. I was lucky to stay out of jail and survive.

At 3:00 A.M. on Tuesday, November 29, 1983, I was puzzled and concerned. I had just spent the evening with my childhood friends Pete and Dennis. Afterward, I asked Pete how I could revitalize my friendship with Dennis. His answer alluded to our different life styles, noting that Dennis had children, worked a 9-to-5 shift and led a much different life than I. Pete urged me to return to Independence Center, the local Fountain House model program, and to seek work through its transitional placement program. There was a conflict here. Pete's advice was inconsistent with my own paranoid world view, but he was one friend who had kept in touch with me, despite some of my bizarre actions over the past 10 years. Pete, my best friend, whom I had met in Cub Scouts in second grade (24 years earlier), was an officer in the Navy, based in Washington, D.C. I was unable to reconcile his involvement in the "government conspiracy" that I assumed with his obvious compassion and superhuman efforts to continue our friendship.

It was during the early morning hours of this day, November 29, 1983, that I, for the first time in 10 years, *considered* the possibility that I was—as those who loved me had told me—insane, and that I had been insane for the past 10 years.

As I lay in bed this night, I remembered back to 1977. During that year, I had been suffering from buzzing sensations in my head, which I became convinced were caused by electricity coming through the floor of my home. In response to this conclusion, I had cut the phone lines and disconnected all of the electric lines in the circuit breaker box in our basement. I realized now, 6 years later, that electricity does not come through the floor of homes. The net result of my 1977 actions had been a 5-month stay at Missouri's maximum-security psychiatric facility, the Biggs Building at the Fulton State Hospital. My memory of those 5 months was not a pleasant one.

As I reflected upon the fact that electricity is not conducted by wood or carpeting, a wave of fear encompassed me. This moment of realization was, in retrospect, the beginning of my recovery, I was able to reason at the time that if I was wrong about this electricity coming through the floor of my home, then I might be wrong about many things.

As I try now to recall the events of that night I recall fear of the most terrifying type imaginable. Was it possible that I had lost my 20s because of an illness? What did people think of me—a 31-year-old man/child, living in a world of delusion and hallucination? Could I possibly pull my life back together? Was there another way out perhaps, and did I want to continue to live, in view of my terrible behavior toward friends, family, and others over the past 10 years?

I finally came to the conclusion that I would try my hardest to proceed from the realization that I had been mentally ill in 1977, and that the "real world" was as it had been prior to 1973. I decided to proceed with my life under that assumption, and to try to ignore all hallucinations. One has to understand that telling myself that the food was not drugged and that I did not live in a police state hardly made those facts a reality. The voices that I heard inside my head for 10 years continued. My paranoia continued to surface, and I constantly had to fight within my mind to retain my equilibrium of thought and my new world view.

At about 5:00 that morning, I decided to take my friend Pete's advice—to return to Independence Center, and work to get a transitional employment placement. I did so, beginning that day. It was the narrowest of threads, and its development within my mind into the strongest steel cable imaginable was with me as I walked to my mailbox on May 26, 1985.

It is my opinion that too little research has been expended to study the dynamics of recovery from major mental illnesses. It would seem that we spend billions of dollars to ameliorate episodic crises through inpatient treatment, but that we have few or no resources earmarked to study recovery.

My most profound problem during my recovery was what I now call "social retardation." I was 31 years old, and had been ill for 10 years. I had not experienced 10 years of life. My friends, and siblings were married, with good jobs and children. I had not had a serious relationship with a woman for 11 years. I had never held a job for longer than 6 months. Although my mother had forced me to learn to cook and clean, I had, for all intents and purposes, lived with a parent (or parents) for 30 of my 31 years.

I was fortunate, during my 1½ years of recovery, to have the resources of Independence Center (the Fountain House model project located in St. Louis) available to me. From November 1983 to April 1985, this agency provided resources to me that included an apartment; two transitional employment placements, with primarily clerical duties, at which I worked in the morning while returning to the agency in the afternoon to continue my involvement in day treatment activities; the opportunity to become involved in managing the members' financial accounts within the agency (a positive confidence builder related to trust); and assistance in the procurement of state vocational rehabilitation funds to return to school to pursue a social work degree.

From late December 1983 to January 1984, my days typically went as follows: work from 8:30 A.M. to 12:30 P.M., attendance at the center from 1 P.M. to 3 P.M., and the rest if my time spent in my apartment or with friends from the membership at the center. Much of my recovery took place in the apartment where I lived alone. As an aside, many tenets of psychiatric rehabilitation insist that the placement of a mental patient in an apartment alone is contraindicated, and that the provision of a roommate for socialization purposes is essential. I would posit that I would not have recovered with a roommate. My first 6 months of recovery featured a personal battle of the first degree. Many nights were filled with tears of fear and rage—tears over my fear of failing and fear of rejection; tears of rage at the loss of 10 years of my life; tears over some of the things I had done; and tears for the past. Could I have ventilated my feelings with another person present? I doubt it.

Somehow, though, these raging emotions strengthened me. Out of the tears and the fears and the rage came a single-mindedness, consistent with my Scotch–Irish and German forbears, which developed into a stubborn, tunnel-visioned intent to make it. I developed a "me first" attitude, and I was determined to protect my gains at any cost. And I did. If I found myself in a situation that made me uncomfortable, I removed myself. If I found myself around people whose life style revolved around behavior that I thought might put me at risk for decompensation (such as drinking or narcotic use), I removed myself from the situation, the consequences be damned. I lost some friends this way, most of them fellow mental patients, and I wish I could now help them. My priorities in life were getting to work on time every day and maintaining my progress.

The next stage in my recovery revolved around what I have described above as "social retardation." I wanted to date, to become involved in a physical and emotional relationship, but I was scared to death of rejection and the risk that it posed to my recovery. Somehow, I came across the book *I'm OK, You're OK,* and was eventually able to integrate some of its basic tenets into my thought processes (as they related to my desire to facilitate a relationship, without what I felt were the concomitant risks to my then fragile ego). One of the primary tenets of this book is the idea that emotions such as jealousy, anger, and "hurt feelings" are products of the individual person, and not products of those whose actions produce emotions within the individual. I was able to define my feelings as feelings I chose to have, and not as feelings that others elicited from me.

With this philosophy, I was able to deal with many of the feelings I was experiencing. In fact, this process eventually bridged the gap into my work life and my relationships with all friends and family. Instead of being hurt or angered by what I might view as a snub or a lack of confidence by others in my abilities, I was able to cognitively rethink troublesome intrapsychic situations, and either to dispose with them completely as irrelevancies or poor luck, or to reformulate them as goals. A good example of this might be my reaction to a turndown of a date by a "sane" coworker at my transitional job site. My initial reaction was one of hurt and embarrassment, wondering how I could face her the next day. This reaction was consistent with my feelings prior to the onset of my illness in 1973. I instead was able to identify the fact that this woman's turndown was a factor in my life that I could not control, and that I was foolish to let someone else's actions control my emotions. I then chose not to be embarrassed or hurt.

My ability to develop a cognitive method to deal with my feelings was the reason why my recovery continued.

Epilogue

From November 1983 to May 1988, I achieved the following: married my wife, Jacquelyn, and got two stepsons as a bonus; received a bachelor's degree in social work from the University of Missouri–St. Louis; received a master's degree in social work from the George Warren Brown School of Social Work, Washington University, St. Louis; and testified before a subcommittee of the U.S. House of Representatives in regard to protection and advocacy for mentally ill citizens. Finally, I wrote a grant proposal and won funding for the Self-Help Center, a social center employing only current or former mental patients and providing social activities for mentally ill individuals, located in St. Louis County, Missouri.

I will never forget that report card I received in May 1985. I still cry when I think about it. People can and do recover from serious mental illness. There are hundreds of different treatment approaches. Because every patient is different, every patient needs to find the one that works for him or her.

LESSONS LEARNED FROM CONSUMERS

CHAPTER FIFTEEN

Summary, Conclusions, and Implications

Autobiographical accounts provide us with an understanding of the experience of mental illness that we can get in no other way. Although our desire in reporting and discussing patients' statements has been to remain as objective as possible, complete objectivity is probably not possible. We need to take seriously the caution of Estroff and Strauss (1989) that first-person statements are soon transformed by the particular viewpoints about these disorders that we harbor. As these authors say, "The voices of patients are soon drowned out by those of colleagues and theories by conceptual frameworks, and often by invisible assumptions" (p. 323). Burton (1974) expresses a similar concern: He says that it is difficult to be neutral about schizophrenia—to experience it in the way it stands forth in its living and behavioral forms. We tend to impose a framework around it according to our predilections, and this often obscures what a patient is feeling, thinking, and being. We need to put the framework aside for a while.

Estroff and Strauss (1989) have challenged the field to discover and develop methods of inquiry that preserve subjectivity—that protect rather than reduce experiential data. Researchers must learn to deal with the complexities and contradictions that emerge, and to live with the tensions between data and concepts, between formulations and unexpected findings.

It is our belief that it is not possible to listen to patients' statements from a completely naive perspective. We agree with Kelly (1963) that all thinking is based, in part, on prior convictions. What is required of writers, he says, is that they make their prior convictions specific. That is a tall order, and few, if any writers succeed completely in doing so. We have tried to state our orientation in the first few chapters, with coping and adaptation being our essential framework. We believe that essentially all living species are characterized by continual efforts to adapt to, or surmount, barriers in their environments.

We believe with Kelly (1963) that "each person contemplates in his or her own personal way the stream of events upon which he finds himself so swiftly borne" (p. 3). Human beings create their own ways of seeing the world; the world does not create these for them. So it is that our focus is on how mentally ill people see the events in their lives and how this determines the behaviors we observe.

Although a survey of patients' observations does not necessarily result in dramatic changes the way we see mental illnesses, it does illuminate considerably the experiences that people with mental illnesses have. It makes these strange experiences more real to us, thus enhancing our understanding and increasing empathic relationships with patients. An understanding of the way they experience mental illness and the process of change and recovery forms a basis for projecting change in service provision and suggests area for research.

THE EXPERIENCE OF PSYCHOSIS

Disturbed perceptions of the self and the world are the essence of psychosis in mental illness. People with psychotic disorders undergo high levels of stress as they try to accommodate themselves to two realities— that of their inner world and the world as experienced by other people. What is more, their perceived world is often in a state of flux, creating a shifting state of equilibrium to which they are constantly trying to adjust.

Equally traumatic for many of our informants is a sense of loss of self. They recall feeling totally engulfed by their illness during psychotic episodes, as ego boundaries gave way, identity became confused, and outer forces seemed to be in full control. For many, these experiences were terrifying, but for a few patients they had such personal significance that the patients were reluctant to give them up.

Neuroleptic medications are generally effective in reducing or eliminating these more florid symptoms of mental illness, but the sequelae of perceptual dyscontrol or the loss of the sense of self may remain and compound the problem of recovery. After such overwhelming experiences, feelings of being victims of powerful inner and outer forces may persist, leaving individuals feeling unable to influence the course of their lives or the world around them.

A number of other factors in the lives of these people may serve to compound the problem. The illness model of psychiatric disorders may ascribe all undesirable behaviors to the illness, thus asking little of a person by way of initiative, responsibility, and accountability. "Good patients" in hospitals are expected to be passive and compliant, and the role of the staff is to take care of them. Some forms of therapy may augment the sense of victimization, as they lead people to believe that the cause of their difficulties lies in the behavior of others (usually parents), and sometimes in the interactions of members in the family system. When patients can ascribe problems to others, there may be little incentive for them to take control of their own lives.

In spite of the many forces that tend to reaffirm the sense of victimization and helplessness, patients' accounts reveal that they make many efforts in behalf of their own growth and recovery. Some informants remember specific events in their lives, in which they came to realize not only that it was possible to influence the course of their lives, but also that it was incumbent upon them to do so. Such events seem to reaffirm our notion that inherent in being a living person is an active process of striving to overcome difficulties and becoming competent in dealing with the environment. Those who work with the mentally ill must learn to identify and acknowledge the efforts that patients make in the service of their own recovery. Patients may need help in making an accurate appraisal of what they can and cannot influence at a given point in time. Eminent researchers (e.g., Estroff, 1989; Strauss, 1987, 1989a; Strauss et al., 1987; Brier & Strauss, 1983) stress the importance of research regarding the capacity for control and self-direction that is so central to recovery.

Disturbances in thinking have long been considered to be primary disturbances in mental illnesses. Our autobiographical accounts clearly reaffirm this observation. People with schizophrenia and other major mental illnesses report that they suffer disturbances both in content of thought and in the process of thinking. Racing thoughts, thought insertion, loose associations, and disorganized and illogical thinking are frequently reported. Some report slowed thinking, thought blocking, and aphasic kinds of conditions. These impairments have been variously attributed to perceptual disorder, language disturbance, and attentional deficit.

People in the accounts we have examined report very active efforts to cope with their cognitive problems. They have learned to identify and avoid situations that are overstimulating, and to structure their lives and reduce unpredictability. What they cannot prevent by creating a calm and quiet environment, they try to manage by active monitoring and attempting to "purge" obsessive or distracting thoughts. The necessity of providing a low-stress environment through establishing appropriate expectations, creating order and structure, and reducing stimulation and distractions is now understood (or should be understood) by service providers and families and by those who teach them.

Medications tend to alleviate many of the cognitive symptoms of mental illness, but they may not affect cognitive deficits. Stuve, Erickson, and Spaulding (1991) believe that it is important to distinguish between "symptoms" and "deficits." Cognitive symptoms, such as delusions and hallucinations, have long been known in the field of psychiatry. Cognitive deficits include problems of attention, concentration, and memory, and impairments in abstract thinking and concept formation, which often persists even when an individual is stabilized. They have only recently become targets of investigation. "Cognitive rehabilitation" is a term now applied to the use of various techniques to strengthen cognitive functioning. It had its early development in the treatment of traumatic head injury and similar fields, and it has only recently been applied to the field of mental illness. There is a need for considerable research in how to measure cognitive deficits, because some of these deficiencies may be subtle and not readily apparent to even the trained observer. It is possible that some of these deficits precede the onset of illness and could be identified as precursors to it. Research into ways of identifying cognitive deficits and into techniques for remediating them is increasing (Cutting, 1985; Goldberg & Cook, 1990; Stuve et al., 1991; Weiss, 1989).

Patients' statements about emotional experiences and interpersonal relations leave us with less clarity and more ambiguity than statements about many other aspects of major mental illness. The usual understanding is that people with mental illnesses, especially those with schizophrenia, tend to be solitary, unsociable, eccentric, and reclusive. Although observable behaviors may lead one to those conclusions, patients' statements seem to indicate a need for human contact, and some establish very meaningful relationships. Nevertheless, there is evidence that many people with mental illness lead painfully lonely lives—more often as a result of hypersensitivity and lack of skills than of a desire for isolation. Although there may be times during acute phases when individuals are too engrossed in their inner world to relate to others, at other times the need for meaningful relationships is often expressed with great anguish.

Research needs to better establish the nature of the vulnerabilities and barriers that interfere with relatedness. Sometimes these people seem exquisitely sensitive to what others are thinking and feeling, leaving them emotionally overloaded and exhausted. In other cases they seem to have difficulty picking up cues that could help them understand what is going on, and in still others they appear to lack confidence and social skills for appropriate responses. If quality of life is the goal, there is probably no more important area for investigation and program development than this one. Yet we have not found a great deal of research attention to the problem.

Penn (1991) has summarized the literature on social deficits in schizophrenia and concluded that people with schizophrenia have marked impairments in the ability to discriminate accurately among faces and the emotions they express. He feels that such impairments may augment the relapse rate and limit the patients' ability to pick up interpersonal cues in social situations. He also notes that these individuals have difficulty perceiving the emotional/thematic characteristics of an interpersonal situation, which require the inclusion of nonverbal body cues in the stimuli. Penn sees some promise in recent innovative techniques that address cognitive rigidity through training in seeing the world in different ways.

PERCEPTIONS OF CAREGIVING AND TREATMENTS

Although much as been written about the interaction of patients and their families, most of it has been written by professionals. More recently parents have discussed their relationships with mentally ill offspring, but patients themselves have written rather little about the issue; more of their attention has been focused on their inner lives and the history of their illness. When families are mentioned, the statements tend to be brief and, more often than not, positive. This is in sharp contrast to traditional views, which have assumed that families usually play a destructive role in their mentally ill relatives' lives.

Of considerable concern is recent research suggesting that siblings and adult children harbor a range of ambivalent feelings toward a mentally ill family member. They grieve for the ill sibling or parent who has been lost to them; they experience considerable stigma and shame; and they report that their social lives are often seriously compromised. Although parents' experiences with mental illness have been quite well researched, there is still a dearth of information about siblings' and adult children's experiences. Such research is badly needed so that family educators and psychotherapists can begin addressing these problems.

Even though patients' accounts have not contained a great deal about relationships with other family members, it is our belief that the nature of serious mental illnesses is such that they inevitably place a great strain on family relationships. Nancy Chevalier (personal conversation, June 8, 1991) has related with much feeling the strains experienced within her family, in which some members were completely unable to accept the fact that she suffered from a mental illness. She has stressed the importance of professionals' learning to understand the pain of such situations and becoming proficient at helping families heal these wounds.

We believe that many professionals have underestimated the importance of families as support systems to their ill relative. Either because of traditional hostility toward parents or because of a misguided effort to make patients independent of their families, some professionals make little effort to help various family members re-establish the ties so rudely disrupted by the illness. Sometimes the families are dismissed as dysfunctional and the patients are encouraged to develop their own support networks within mental health services. Such professionals underestimate the difficulties many patients have in establishing their own networks, and disregard the possibility that they even more than others, need the continuity and sense of belonging that come with family.

Of considerable interest to us are the attitudes patients have expressed about the quality of care they have received from professional caregivers. Unfortunately, few conclusions can be drawn about the service provider system from these statements, because they vary so considerably. On the negative side, some patients claim that their treatments were totally inappropriate; others report demeaning messages from providers, as well as lack of understanding and ordinary human kindness. However, some patients acknowledge that they also played a role in creating difficult relationships by denying their illness and resisting treatment.

Reactions to professionals are not uniformly negative. Cases have been made for the benefit received in each of the current approaches—hospitalization, medication, psychotherapy, and psychosocial rehabilitation. Trends toward working with patients in more collaborative, less hierarchical relationships have been stressed.

Some patients speak eloquently about the critical importance of a certain therapist in their lives. Coursey (1989) and Zahniser, Coursey, and Hershberger (1991) lament the virtual disappearance of theory and research in the field of psychotherapy in schizophrenia. Coursey believes that it is time that we take a look at new forms of therapy, based on a current understanding of mental illness and its biological basis. He recommends that treatment be "more phenomenologically based, empirically tested and problem-specific" (1989, p. 349).

Coursey (1989) believes that psychotherapy is important in helping clients deal with all the human issues inherent in having a chronic, debilitating disorder. Therapy should deal with the meanings and understandings that persons have about themselves and the world around them. It should help them see themselves more accurately and help them come to terms cognitively and emotionally with their situation. It should help them come to terms with their injured selves, develop an acceptable identity, and find meaning and purpose in life.

Psychiatric rehabilitation is an important but relatively new form of treatment that has gained wide acceptance in mental illness (Anthony & Liberman, 1986; Liberman, 1986). Few of our informants have specifically commented on experiences with rehabilitation — probably because it is not universally available. All three consumers who have written chapters for this book, however, share exceptionally positive experiences in such programs. The views of others are less positive, and a recent study (Hatfield, 1989) using families as informants suggested significant criticism of programs as they are now implemented. These families questioned the lack of program diversity to meet individual needs, as well as failure to consider compatibility in age and functionality in grouping people. They felt that some programs were demeaning and boring.

The profession of psychosocial rehabilitation seems to have taken a fairly strong behavioral direction in its early years. Perhaps now that we are beginning to better understand the experiential side of mental illness, more attention will be given to the experience of mental illness from the ill persons' perspective. This will enable practioners to develop more empathic relationships with clients and to enhance their capacity to offer more support and guidance on such difficult questions as meaning, identity, and purpose in life.

There has been a commendable tendency in rehabilitation to place a strong emphasis on the strengths of people with mental illnesses. However, this seems to have led to discounting the very real cognitive impairments many of these people face. With greater sophistication in assessing cognitive impairment and in modifying learning experiences for individual learning styles, it is conceivable that individuals may make more significant gains in knowledge and skills. In addition, recent developments in cognitive rehabilitation may make it possible for us to improve cognitive processes, or the ways that people reason and think.

Finally, we must acknowledge that the interpersonal environment extends much further than the family or the service provider system. Since most mentally ill people now live in the community, how well they do depends to a large extent on the supportiveness of that larger community — and, of course, the larger community is a much harder one to influence. Most patients report that they have not been well accepted by others in the community. On the contrary, they feel rejected, stigmatized, and discriminated against in work, housing, and peer relationships. The consequences to such individuals are enormous. Stigma produces self-hatred and rejection of mentally ill peers. It causes people to deny their illnesses, and thus to fail to get appropriate treatments; it also causes many people to take on strange defensive postures, which aggravate social unacceptability. Stigma is a source of endless suffering, and it serves as a great barrier to people's getting better.

Research studies on stigma tend to confirm that there is considerable negative feeling against people with mental illnesses. Such studies now need to address the various reasons for rejection. It is probable that the way mentally ill people are perceived and what is seen as objectionable about them may differ considerably, depending upon the persons we are talking to. We need to understand these various perceptions of the mentally ill, so that we can design programs to address the problem more accurately. The issue of stigma is not new to the field of social science. Social scientists have studied stigma as it relates to other social problems (e.g., racism, poverty, illegitimacy, etc.); the findings in these areas could offer insights about stigma in mental illness.

PERCEPTIONS OF
THE RECOVERY PROCESS

In Chapter 11 we have discussed some of the varying concepts of recovery and concluded that the use of the word "recovery" in a major mental illness does not usually mean "cure" or return to the premorbid state. Rather, it means a kind of readaptation to the illness that allows life to go forward in a meaningful way. The adaptive response is not an end state; it is a process by which the person is continually trying to maximize the fit between his or her needs and the environment.

The autobiographical accounts we have examined, and the work of such authorities as Strauss (1989a), suggest that efforts at healing may go on continually even when a person appears to be experiencing a plateau in improvement. People go through periods of organization followed by periods of disorganization. A person may seem to be getting worse or more ill during a period of disorganization, but important changes may be occurring in attitudes, perception, and meaning, and these may eventually result in higher levels of growth. We need longitudinal studies to help us see patterns in a person's life.

Patients speak most often of their acceptance of the illness, the maintenance of a hopeful attitude, and having the right kind of support as the most important factors in their recovery. Although it is certain that most professionals and families also place great emphasis on the need for acceptance, we have found a growing interest expressed in the professional literature in understanding what we mean by "acceptance" and the kinds of psychological mechanisms various individuals use to achieve it. It is important to know whether an individual's acceptance occurs through resignation, compromise, change of goals, or something else, and how self-esteem and sense of control are affected.

Some of the most poignant statements made by patients have to do with the experience of hope. Little can be accomplished without hope; yet we know little about the way professionals and families can be effective in instilling hope. Patients say that they need people who believe in them, who hold appropriate expectations for them, and who are able to observe and articulate the strengths they have manifested in their struggles to survive the ravages of their illnesses.

Of critical importance to patients in the process of getting better is the quality of affection and support that others give. Most often mentioned by patients are informal relationships and friends. Some have found these kinds of relationships in the former-patient subculture and in drop-in centers, where they have learned the satisfaction of both giving and receiving support. Others have found support in special relationships with caring professionals in whom they have developed trust and confidence.

What matters in the last analysis is how these individuals come to see themselves and their place in the world. Although growing up and establishing a satisfactory personal identity are difficult for most young adults, the barriers that our informants have faced and continue to face are enormous. Barriers lie both in the devastating consequences of the illness to an individual's development and in the social rejection and stigma that are inevitably encountered.

The nature of the psychotic experience is such that individuals may lose their sense of self and of their place in the world for long periods of time. Experiences become fragmented and distorted, and attempts to negotiate both inner and outer realities are overwhelming challenges. Even when patients are stabilized, it may be difficult for them to know which past experiences were real and which were a part of the psychotic experience. Long periods of patienthood do not provide an identity that is valued and respected in the wider world; yet many persons with highly chronic conditions know no other identity than that of patient. The challenge to professionals is to help these individuals see themselves as something other than mental patients. This requires the ability to see their unique characteristics and to help them see themselves as unique and interesting.

The formation of an identity is based partly on how others in the community regard one. Social rejection is so pervasive that few people with a mental illness are untouched by it. Patients' personal accounts are replete with statements of the demoralization they experience when they are socially devalued because of something they cannot help. As we have already noted, we believe that the reasons for social rejection are more complex than they are ordinarily depicted in the literature, and that we need to rethink the way in which the problem is conceptualized so that more effective antistigma programs can be developed.

In spite of these formidable barriers, however, it is heartening to note that many of our informants have found ways to create meaning in their lives. They have done this in the way common to most people—by developing a sense of accomplishment and a sense of usefulness to others that are compatible with their present circumstances. They took great pride in learning to understand their illnesses and in developing strategies for controlling the symptoms and staying stable. Although many feel that having a regular job is their greatest ambition, others take satisfaction in accomplishments in hobbies, the arts, and physical fitness. A number of people feel that their ability to manage their own illnesses has made them especially suited to become "wounded healers" to others beginning the struggle. Clearly, there is no greater challenge for a caring society than to identify and support meaningful roles for those who are unable to do competitive work.

The cyclical nature of these disorders complicates enormously the problem of establishing new identities, new purposes, and new meanings to life. The gains that have been made are constantly threatened by a re-emergence of symptoms and the resulting possibilities of decompensation, rehospitalization, and having to start over again. As one patient has so aptly stated it, it is much like the experience of Sisyphus, who according to legend succeeds in rolling a huge boulder up a mountain again and again, only to have it roll once more to the bottom.

Given the unpredictable course of the illness, many patients have learned to identify the symptoms that point to potential relapse and to make a timely intervention. The signals of potential trouble vary with individuals—sleeplessness, fatigue, difficulty in concentration, eating less, hypersensitivity, tension, and increased hallucinations and delusions, to name a few of the more common ones. Gaining this kind of awareness takes time and often occurs only after many serious setbacks.

Recognizing the symptoms is one thing, but learning appropriate responses is another. Some people have learned to withdraw from overstimulating environments; others seek support from friends or family members; and still others turn to their doctors for medication adjustments. Although many patients quoted in this book have learned to make these adaptive responses, we know of others who seem not to learn and continue to be at the mercy of their disorders.

Although many patients do a remarkable job of managing their symptoms, the role of the mental health system continues to be important. Hospitals and clinics increasingly offer training sessions to patients about their illnesses, ways to become alert to symptoms, and steps they should take. Unfortunately, this sensible approach is a rather recent development in treatment and is not yet available everywhere.

THOUGHTS ON FUTURE DIRECTIONS

For a number of years, Rutter (1986) has called for studies of that large population of individuals who do not become psychiatrically ill, despite being subject to the genetic and life stress variables that appear to be related to major psychiatric illnesses in other individuals. Sabshin (1990) states:

> By the beginning of the twenty-first century, I believe that the adaptability of many individuals with apparent high-risk loading for psychiatric illness will not be able to be ignored. . . . The psychobiology of coping and adaptability will become a major part of psychiatric research and practice. Integral to this new emphasis will be the transactions and interactions between psychological adaptation and biological systems. (pp. 1272–1273)

Investigations of these patterns in normal populations—attempts to distinguish why some people become ill and some do not—have their analogues in populations of persons with diagnosed psychopathology. Why do some persons with histories of multiple hospitalizations and clear disability become better, while others do not? We see evidence of unexpected improvements not only in longitudinal research (Ciompi, 1980; Harding, Brooks, Ashikaga, Strauss, & Breier, 1987), but also in the personal histories of former patients now active in the consumer movement, some of whose recollections are provided in this book. The major question for the coming century is to what extent this improvement can be brought about by timely interventions—by understanding the interrelationships of biological, psychological, sociocultural, and other environmental variables, and learning to work at their interface in highly specific ways.

We must take it as a given that flexibility exists in schizophrenia as well as in other major mental illnesses. Although this flexibility may be limited by the nature of the disease, a patient nevertheless has a coping self that is responsive to positive stimuli and open to change. The sensitive, caring clinician can permeate this boundary, typically through empathic listening and supportive psychotherapy, which helps the patient process his or her experience of the disease and its consequences. The caring family provides the bedrock to which the person can always turn for continuity, support, and most of all, a sense of permanent commitment to his or her welfare.

Research that focuses only on treatment models or the mediating role of support systems, however, tends to ignore the specific strengths that enable individuals to respond, benefit, and grow. We need continuing research on patients' phenomenological and interpersonal experiences, as well as more refined measures for ascertaining critical coping strategies. We need to empower the patients themselves to provide the answers. Let us hope that their personal accounts will help us develop the right questions and the right methodology to enlighten the field as to why and how people are able to get better.

References

Abraham, D. (1982). We have a dream. In H. Shetler & P. Straw (Eds.), *A new day: Voices from across the land* (pp. 30–31). Arlington, VA: National Alliance for the Mentally Ill.

American Psychiatric Association. (1987). *Diagnostic and statistical manual of mental disorders* (3rd ed., rev.). Washington, DC: Author.

Anderson, C. M., Reiss, D. J., & Hogarty, G. E. (1986). *Schizophrenia and the family: A practitioner's guide to psychoeducation and management.* New York: Guilford Press.

Andreasen, N., & Grove, W. (1986). Thought, language, and communication in schizophrenia: Diagnosis and prognosis. *Schizophrenia Bulletin, 12,* 348–359.

Anonymous. (1955). An autobiography of a schizophrenic experience. *Journal of Abnormal and Social Psychology, 51,* 667–687.

Anonymous. (1989a). After the funny farm. In National Alliance for the Mentally Ill, *The experiences of patients and families: First person accounts reprinted from Schizophrenia Bulletin and the New York Times* (pp. 1–3). Arlington, VA: NAMI.

Anonymous. (1989b). Maintaining health in a turbulent world. In National Alliance for the Mentally Ill, *The experiences of patients and families: First person accounts reprinted from Schizophrenia Bulletin and the New York Times* (pp. 17–21). Arlington, VA: NAMI.

Anonymous. (1989c). Problems of living with schizophrenia. In National Alliance for the Mentally Ill, *The experiences of patients and families: First person accounts reprinted from Schizophrenia Bulletin and the New York Times* (pp. 4–5). Arlington VA: NAMI.

Anonymous. (1989d). The quiet discrimination. In National Alliance for the Mentally Ill, *The experiences of patients and families: First person accounts reprinted from Schizophrenia Bulletin and the New York Times* (pp. 14–16). Arlington, VA: NAMI.

Anscombe, R. (1987). The disorder of consciousness in schizophrenia. *Schizophrenia Bulletin, 13,* 221–260.

Anthony, E. J., & Cohler, B. J. (Eds.) (1987). *The invulnerable child*. New York: Guilford Press.

Anthony, W. A., & Liberman, R. P. (1986). The practice of psychiatric rehabilitation: Historical, conceptual, and research base. *Schizophrenia Bulletin, 12,* 542–559.

Antonovsky, A. (1979). *Health, stress, and coping*. San Francisco: Jossey-Bass.

Arieti, S. (1981). The family of the schizophrenic and its participation in the therapeutic task. In S. Arieti & K. H. Brodie (Eds.), *American handbook of psychiatry* (2nd ed., Vol. 7, pp. 271–284). New York: Basic Books.

Bachrach, L. L. (1986). Conceptual issues: The questions that precede the research questions. In J. P. Bowker & A. Rubin (Eds.), *Studies on chronic mental illness: New horizons for social work researchers* (pp. 29–51). Washington, DC: Council on Social Work Education.

Bachrach. L. L. (1988). Defining chronic mental illness: A concept paper. *Hospital and Community Psychiatry, 39,* 383–388.

Barbera, D. (1982). Pet peeves. In H. Shetler & P. Straw (Eds.), *A new day: Voices from across the land* (pp. 25–26). Arlington, VA: National Alliance for the Mentally Ill.

Barrett, R. J, (1989). Interpretations of schizophrenia. *Culture, Medicine and Psychiatry, 12,* 357–388.

Beck, A. T., Rush, A. J., Shaw, B. F., & Emery, G. (1979). *Cognitive therapy of depression*. New York: Guilford Press.

Benjamin, L. S. (1989). Is chronicity a function of the relationship between the person and the auditory hallucination? *Schizophrenia Bulletin, 15,* 291–310.

Bennet, G. (1979). *Patients and their doctors: The journey through medical care*. London: Bailliere, Tindall.

Bernheim, K., & Lehman, A. (1985). *Working with families of the mentally ill*. New York: Norton.

Bernheim, K., Lewine, R., & Beale, C. T. (1982). *The caring family*. New York: Random House.

Blanch, A. (1990). *Report on Roundtable on Alternatives to Involuntary Treatment, September 14–15, 1990, Bethesda, MD*. Unpublished manuscript, Community Support Program, National Institute of Mental Health.

Blaska, B. (1991). First person account: What it is like to be treated like a CMI. *Schizophrenia Bulletin, 17,* 173–176.

Bleuler, E. (1950). *Dementia praecox or the group of schizophrenias*. New York: International Universities Press. (Original work published 1911)

Bockes, Z. (1989). "Freedom" means knowing you have a choice. In National Alliance for the Mentally Ill, *The experiences of patients and families: First person accounts reprinted from Schizophrenia Bulletin and the New York Times* (pp. 40–42). Arlington VA: NAMI.

Borgeson, N. (1982). Schizophrenia from the inside. In H. Shetler & P. Straw (Eds.), *A new day: Voices from across the land* (pp. 6–8). Arlington, VA: National Alliance for the Mentally Ill.

Bouricius, J. K. (1989). Negative symptoms and emotions in schizophrenia. *Schizophrenia Bulletin, 15,* 201–208.

Brier, A., & Strauss, J. (1983). Self control in psychotic disorders. *Archives of General Psychiatry, 40,* 1141–1145.

Brodoff, A. S. (1988). First person account: Schizophrenia through a sister's eyes—the burden of invisible baggage. *Schizophrenia Bulletin, 14,* 113–116.

Brundage, B. E. (1983). What I wanted to know but was afraid to ask. *Schizophrenia Bulletin, 9,* 584–586.

Buie, J. (1989, October). Psychologist prevails despite schizophrenia. *APA Monitor,* p. 23.

Burton, A. (1974). Preface. In A. Button, J. Lopez-Ibor, & W. Mendel (Eds.), *Schizophrenia as a life style* (pp. xiii–xiv). New York: Springer.

Cameron, N. (1944). Experimental analysis of schizophrenic thinking. In J. S. Kasanin (Ed.), *Language and thought in schizophrenia.* New York: Norton.

Campbell, J. (Ed.). (1989a). *The Well-Being Project: Mental health clients speak for themselves* (California Department of Mental Health, In Pursuit of Wellness, Vol. 6). Sacramento: The California Network of Mental Health Clients.

Campbell, J. (Ed.). (1989b). *People say I'm crazy: An anthology of art, poetry, prose, photography and testimony by mental health clients throughout California.* Sacramento: California Department of Mental Health.

Canadian Mental Health Association. (1985). *Building a framework for support for people with severe mental disabilities: Listening.* Toronto: Author.

Caplan, G. (1974). *Support systems and community mental health.* New York: Behavioral Publications.

Caplan, P. J., & Hall-McCorquodale, I. (1985). The scapegoating of mothers: A call for change. *American Journal of Orthopsychiatry, 55,* 610–613.

Carpenter, W. T. (1986). Thoughts on the treatment of schizophrenia. *Schizophrenia Bulletin, 12,* 527–539.

Carpenter, W. T., & Hanlon, T. (1986). Clinical practice and the phenomenology of schizophrenia. In G. Burrows, T. Norman, & G. Rubinstein (Eds.), *Handbook of studies on schizophrenia* (pp. 123–130). New York: Elsevier.

Carver, C. S., Scheier, M. F., & Weintraub, J. K. (1989). Assessing coping strategies: A theoretically based approach. *Journal of Personality and Social Psychology, 56,* 267–283.

Chamberlin, J. (1978). *On our own: Patient controlled alternatives to the mental health system.* New York: McGraw-Hill.

Chevalier, N. Y. (1990, January 16). When pills, shock therapy failed . . . I imagined dancing in Vienna. *The Washington Post,* Health section, pp. 12–14.

Ciompi, L. (1980). Catamnestic long-term study of the course of life and aging of schizophrenics. *Schizophrenia Bulletin, 6,* 606–616.

Clarkin, J. F., & Haas, G. L. (1988). Assessment of affective disorders and their interpersonal contexts. In J. F. Clarkin, G. L. Haas, & I. D. Glick (Eds.), *Affective disorders and the family: Assessment and treatment* (pp. 29–50). New York: Guilford Press.

Clausen, J. A. (1980). The family, stigma, and help-seeking in severe mental disorders. In J. G. Rabkin, L. Gelb, & J. B. Lazar (Eds.), *Attitudes toward the mentally ill: Research perspectives* (pp. 31–34). Washington, DC: U. S. Government Printing Office.

Corbett, L. (1976). Perceptual dyscontrol: A possible organizing principle for schizophrenia research. *Schizophrenia Bulletin, 2,* 249–265.

Corrigan, P. W., Davies-Farmer, R. M., & Lome, H. B. (1988). A curriculum-based psychoeducational program for the mentally ill. *Psychosocial Rehabilitation Journal, 12* (2), 71–73.

Corrigan, P. W., Liberman, R. P., & Engel, J. D. (1990). From noncompliance to collaboration in the treatment of schizophrenia. *Hospital and Community Psychiatry, 41,* 1203–1211.

Coursey, R. (1989). Psychotherapy with persons suffering from schizophrenia: The need for a new agenda. *Schizophrenia Bulletin, 15,* 349–354.

Cutting, J. (1985). *The psychology of schizophrenia.* New York: Churchill Livingstone.

Day, R., Nielsen, A., Korten, A., Ernberg, G., Dube, K. C., Gebhart, J., Jeblensky, A., Leon, C., Marsella, A., Olatawura, M., Sartorius, N., Strömgren, E., Takahashi, R., Wig, N., & Wynne, L. C. (1987). Stressful life events preceding the acute onset of schizophrenia: A cross-national study from the World Health Organization. *Culture, Medicine and Psychiatry, 11,* 123–205.

Dearth, N., Labenski, B. J., Mott, M. E., & Pelligrini, L. M. (1986). *Families helping families: Living with schizophrenia.* New York: Norton.

Deegan, P. E. (1988). Recovery: The lived experience of rehabilitation. *Psychosocial Rehabilitation Journal, 11* (4), 11–19.

DeVries, M., & Delespaul, P. (1989). Time, context, and subjective experiences in schizophrenia. *Schizophrenia Bulletin, 15,* 233–244.

Doughty, J. (1987, January). Woman tells of battle with schizophrenia. *Quarterly Newsletter of Families and Friends Alliance for the Mentally Ill,* p. 3, Lafayette, LA.

Eaton, W. W. (1986). *The sociology of mental disorders* (2nd ed.). New York: Praeger.

Eckman, T. A., Liberman, R. P., & Phipps, C. C. (1990). Teaching medication management skills to schizophrenic patients. *Journal of Clinical Psychopharmacology, 10,* 33–38.

Emerick, R. (1990). Self-help groups for former patients: Relations with mental health professionals. *Hospital and Community Psychiatry, 41,* 401–407.

Erikson, E. (1968). *Identity: Youth and crisis.* New York: Norton.

Estroff, S. E. (1981). *Making it crazy: An ethnography of psychiatric clients in an American community.* Berkeley: University of California Press.

Estroff, S. E. (1989). Self, identity, and subjective experiences of schizophrenia: In search of the subject. *Schizophrenia Bulletin, 15,* 323–324.

Fabrega, H. (1989). The self and schizophrenia: A cultural perspective. *Schizophrenia Bulletin, 15,* 277–290.

Falloon, I. R. H. , Boyd, J. L. & McGill, C. W. (1984). *Family care of schizophrenia.* New York: Guilford Press.

Feldman, D. (1974). Chronic disabling illness: A holistic view. *Journal of Chronic Disease, 27,* 287–291.

Fish, G. (1985, September). What it's like to be chronically depressed. *Indiana Community Support System Network News,* p. 2.

Freedman, M. A. (1974). Subjective experiences of perceptual and cognitive disturbances in schizophrenia. *Archives of General Psychiatry, 30,* 333–340.

Gara, M., Rosenberg, S., & Mueller, D. (1989). Perceptions of self and others in schizophrenia. *International Journal of Personal Construct Psychology, 2,* 253–270.

George, A. L. (1974). Adaptation to stress in political decision making: The individual, small group, and organizational contexts. In. G. V. Coelho, D. A. Hamburg. & J. E. Adams (Eds.), *Coping and adaptation* (pp. 176–245). New York: Basic Books.

Godschalx, S. M. (1987). *Experiences and coping strategies of people with schizophrenia.* Unpublished doctoral dissertation, University of Utah.

Goffman, E. (1961). *Asylums.* Chicago: Aldine.

Goldberg, J. O., & Cooke, P. E. (1990, July). *Cognitive rehabilitation and schizophrenia.* Paper presented at an International Conference organized by the British Columbia Mental Health Society, Vancouver.

Greenfield, D., Strauss, J. S., Bowers, M. B., & Mandelkern, M. (1989). Insight and interpretation of illness on recovery from psychosis. *Schizophrenia Bulletin, 15,* 245–252.

Harding, C. M., Brooks, G., Ashikaga, T. Strauss, J. S., & Breier, A. (1987). The Vermont Longitudinal Study of persons with severe mental illness: II. Long-term outcome of subjects who retrospectively met DSM-III criteria for schizophrenia. *American Journal of Psychiatry, 144,* 727–735.

Harding, C. M., Zubin, J. & Strauss, J. S. (1987). Chronicity in schizophrenia: Fact, partial fact, or artifact. *Hospital and Community Psychiatry, 38,* 477–485.

Harris, M., & Bergman, H, (1984). The young adult chronic patient: Affective responses to treatment. In B. Pepper & H. Ryglewicz (Eds.), *New directions for mental health services: No. 21. Advances in treating the young adult chronic patient* (pp. 29–36). San Francisco: Jossey-Bass.

Hatfield, A. B. (1987a). Coping and adaption: A conceptual framework for understanding families. In A. B. Hatfield & H. P. Lefley (Eds.), *Families of the mentally ill: Coping and adaptation* (pp. 60–84). New York: Guilford Press.

Hatfield, A. B. (1987b). Social supports and family coping. In A. B. Hatfield & H. P. Lefley (Eds.), *Families of the mentally ill: Coping and adaptation* (pp. 191–207). Guilford Press.

Hatfield, A. B. (1989). Serving the unserved in community rehabilitation programs. *Psychosocial Rehabilitation Journal, 13,* 71–77.

Hatfield, A. B. (1990). *Family education in mental illness.* New York: Guilford Press.

Hatfield, A. B., & Lefley, H. P. (Eds.). (1987). *Families of the mentally ill: Coping and adaptation.* New York: Guilford Press.

Hatfield, A. B., Spaniol, L. & Zipple, A. M. (1987). Expressed emotion: A family perspective. *Schizophrenia Bulletin, 13,* 221–226.

Herz, M. I. (1984). Recognizing and preventing relapse in patients with schizophrenia. *Hospital and Community Psychiatry, 35,* 344–349.

Herz, M. I., & Melville, C. (1980). Relapse in schizophrenia. *American Journal of Psychiatry, 137,* 801–805.

Hirsch, S. R., & Leff, J. P. (1975). *Abnormalities in parents of schizophrenics.* London: Oxford University Press.

Holmes, D. S. (1991). *Abnormal psychology.* New York: Harper Collins.

Holmes, T. H. , & Rahe, R. H. (1967). The Social Readjustment Rating Scale. *Journal of Psychosomatic Research, 11,* 213–218.

Holzman, P., Shenton, M., & Solovay, M. (1986). Quality of thought disorder in differential diagnosis. *Archives of General Psychiatry, 12,* 360–372.

Houghton, J. F. (1982). Maintaining mental health in a turbulent world. *Schizophrenia Bulletin, 8,* 548–549.

Howells, J. G., & Guirguis, W. R. (1985). *The family and schizophrenia.* New York: International Universities Press.

Hudson, W. (1974). Strike another match. In *Madness Network News Reader* (pp. 53–55). San Francisco: Glide.

Irvine, C. L. (1985). *Coping successfully with mental and emotional disorders: Five personal success stories.* Unpublished mimeograph, Alliance for the Mentally Ill of Marin County, CA.

Isaac, R. J., & Armat, V. C. (1990). *Madness in the streets: How psychiatry and the law abandoned the mentally ill.* New York: Free Press.

Janacek, J. (1991, May 17). Residential housing [Letter to the editor]. *Psychiatric News,* p. 16.

Johnston, M., & Holtzman, P. (1979). *Assessing schizophrenic thinking.* San Francisco: Jossey-Bass.

Jones, M. (1975). Community care for chronic mental patients: The need for reassessment. *Hospital and Community Psychiatry, 26,* 423–427.

Kanter, J. S. (1985). Moral issues and mental illness. In J. S. Kanter (Ed.), *New directions for mental health services: No. 27. Clinical issues in treating the chronic mentally ill* (pp. 47–62). San Francisco: Jossey-Bass.

Kanter, J. S., Lamb. H. R., & Loeper, C. (1987). Expressed emotion in families: A critical review. *Hospital and Community Psychiatry, 38,* 374–380.

Kaplan, B. (Ed.). (1964). *The inner world of mental illness: A series of first person accounts of what it was like.* New York: Harper & Row.

Keil, J. (1984). *Overcoming the recurring nightmare of schizophrenia.* San Diego: K. & A.

Kelley, H. H., & Michela, J. (1980). Attribution theory and research. *Annual Review of Psychology, 31,* 457–501.

Kelly, G. (1963). *A theory of personality: The psychology of personal constructs.* New York: Norton Press.

Kerlinger, F. N. (1973). *Foundations of behavioral research* (2nd ed.). New York: Holt, Rinehart & Winston.

Kersker, S. (1990, December). Comments. *AMI News: Alliance for the Mentally Ill of St. Petersburg and Clearwater, FL,* p. 2.

King-Hasher, C. (1989, Fall). Full circle. *Journal of the California Alliance for the Mentally Ill,* pp. 8–9.

Kytle, E. R. (1987). *The voices of Robby Wilde.* Washington, DC: Seven Locks Press.

Lally, S. J. (1989). Does being in here mean something is wrong with me? *Schizophrenia Bulletin, 15,* 253–265.

Lamb, R. (1982). The young adult chronic patients: The new drifters. *Hospital and Community Psychiatry, 33,* 465–468.

Landis, C. & Mettler, F. (1964). *Varieties of psychopathological experience.* New York: Holt, Rinehart & Winston.

Lanquetot, R. (1984). First person account: Confessions of the daughter of a schizophrenic. *Schizophrenia Bulletin, 10,* 467–471.

Lazarus, R. S. (1966). *Psychological stress and the coping process.* New York: McGraw-Hill.

Lazarus, R. S., & Folkman, S. (1984). *Stress, appraisal, and coping.* New York: Springer.

Leete, E. (1982). Overcoming the stigma of mental illness. In H. Shetler & P. Straw (Ed.), *A new day: Voices from across the land* (pp. 3–5). Arlington, VA: National Alliance for the Mentally Ill.

Leete, E. (1987a). A patient's perspective on schizophrenia. In A. B. Hatfield (Ed.), *New directions for mental health services: No. 34. Families of the mentally ill: Meeting the challenges* (pp. 81–90). San Francisco: Jossey-Bass.

Leete, E. (1987b). The treatment of schizophrenia: A patient's perspective. *Hospital and Community Psychiatry, 38,* 486–491.

Leete, E. (1988). A consumer perspective on psychosocial treatment. *Psychosocial Rehabilitation Journal, 12* (2), 45–62.

Leete, E. (1989). How I perceive and manage my illness. *Schizophrenia Bulletin, 15,* 197–200.

Leff, J. P., & Vaughn, C. E. (1985). *Expressed emotion in families.* New York: Guilford Press.

Lefley, H. P. (1984). Delivering mental health services across cultures. In P. B. Pedersen, N. Sartorius, & A. M. Marsella (Eds.), *Mental health services: The cultural context* (pp. 135–171). New York: Sage.

Lefley, H. P. (1987). Culture and mental illness: The family role. In A. B. Hatfield & H. P. Lefley (Eds.), *Families of the mentally ill: Coping and adaptation* (pp. 30–59). New York: Guilford Press.

Lefley, H. P. (1990). Culture and chronic mental illness. *Hospital and Community Psychiatry, 41,* 277–286.

Lefley, H. P. (1992). Expressed emotion: Conceptual, clinical, and social policy implications. *Hospital and Community Psychiatry, 43,* 591–598.

Lefley, H. P., & Johnson, D. L. (Eds.). (1990). *Families as allies in treatment of the mentally ill: New directions for mental health professionals.* Washington DC; American Psychiatric Press.

Leggatt, M. (1986). Schizophrenia: The consumer viewpoint. In A. Burrows, T. Norman, & G. Rubenstein (Eds.), *Handbook of studies of schizophrenia* (Part 2, pp. 143–153). New York: Elsevier.

Lehman, A. (1982). The well-being of chronic mental patients. *Archives of General Psychiatry, 40,* 369–373.

Lehman, A. (1982). A quality of life interview. *Evaluation and Program Planning, 11,* 52–62.

Liberman, R. P. (1986). Psychiatric rehabilitation of schizophrenia: Editor's introduction. *Schizophrenia Bulletin, 12,* 540–541.

Liberman, R. P. (1987). *Psychiatric rehabilitation of chronic mental patients.* Washington, DC: American Psychiatric Press.

Liberman, R. P., Mueser, K., Wallace, C. J., Jacobs, H. E., Eckman, T., & Massel, H. K. (1986). Training skills in the psychiatrically disabled: Learning coping and competence. *Schizophrenia Bulletin, 12,* 631–646.

Liem, J. H. (1980). Family studies of schizophrenia: An update and commentary. *Schizophrenia Bulletin, 6,* 429–455.

Lin, K. M., & Kleinman, A. M. (1988). Psychopathology and clinical course of schizophrenia: A cross-cultural perspective. *Schizophrenia Bulletin, 14,* 555–567.

Link, B. G. (1991, Winter). Overcoming stigma: A powerful influence on people's lives. *National Alliance for the Mentally Ill, Decade of the Brain,* pp. 4–6.

Loder, A. (1991, June). *Perspectives on managed care in the public sector.* Paper presented at the 40th National Conference on Mental Health Statistics, National Institute of Mental Health, Washington, DC.

Lovejoy, M. (1989). Expectations and the recovery process. In National Alliance for the Mentally Ill, *The experiences of patients and families: First person accounts reprinted from Schizophrenia Bulletin and the New York Times* (pp. 23–27). Arlington, VA: NAMI.

MacDonald, N. (1960). The other side: Living with schizophrenia. *Canadian Medical Association Journal, 82,* 218–221.

MacKinnon, B. L. (1977). Psychiatric depression and the need for significance. *American Journal of Psychiatry, 134,* 427–429.

McFarlane, W. R., & Beels, C. C. (1983). Family research in schizophrenia: A review and integration for clinicians. In W. R. MacFarlane (Ed.), *Family therapy in schizophrenia* (pp. 311–323). New York: Guilford Press.

McGhie, A., & Chapman, J, (1961). Disorders of attention and perception in early schizophrenia. *Psychology, 34,* 103–116.

McGlashan, T., & Carpenter, W. (1976). Post-psychotic depression schizophrenia. *Archives of General Psychiatry, 33,* 231–239.

McGlashan, T., Levy, S. & Carpenter, W. (1975). Integration and sealing over. *Archives of General Psychiatry, 32,* 1269–1272.

McGrath, M. (1984). First person account: Where did I go? *Schizophrenia Bulletin, 10,* 638–640.

McKenzie, C. (1982). Recovery. In H. Shetler & P. Straw (Eds.), *A new day: Voices from across the land* (pp. 18–20). Arlington, VA: National Alliance for the Mentally Ill.

Mechanic, D. (1974). Social structure and personal adaptation: Some neglected dimensions. In G. V. Coelho, D. A. Hamburg, & J. E. Adams (Eds.), *Coping and adaptation* (pp. 32–44). New York: Basic Books.

Mechanic, D. (1984). Sociocultural and social-psychological factors affecting personal responses to psychological disorder. In J. E. Mezzich & C. E. Berganza (Eds.), *Culture and psychopathology* (pp. 443–460). New York: Columbia University Press.

Mendel, W. (1974). A phenomenological theory of schizophrenia. In A. Burton, J. Lopez-Obor, & W. Mendel (Eds.), *Schizophrenia as a life style* (pp. 106–155). New York: Springer.

Minkoff, K., & Stern, R. (1985). Paradoxes faced by residents being trained in the psychosocial treatment of people with chronic schizophrenia. *Hospital and Community Psychiatry, 36,* 859–864.

Minor, D. (1989). Third side of the coin. In National Alliance for the Mentally Ill, *The experiences of patients and families: First person accounts reprinted from Schizophrenia Bulletin and the New York Times.* Arlington, VA: NAMI.

Monat, A., & Lazarus, R. S. (1977). *Stress and coping.* New York: Columbia University Press.

Moorman, M. (1988, September 11). A sister's need. *New York Times Magazine,* pp. 44, 46, 50, 52, 53, 116.

Nasrallah, H. A., & Weinberger, D. R. (1986). *The neurology of schizophrenia.* New York: Elsevier.

National Alliance for the Mentally Ill. (1989). *The experiences of patients and families: First person accounts reprinted from Schizophrenia Bulletin and the New York Times.* Arlington, VA: Author.

Newman, E. (1989, July). God bless the ground. *Arkansas Alliance for the Mentally Ill Newsletter,* p. 3.

North, C. (1987). *Welcome silence: My triumph over schizophrenia.* New York: Simon & Schuster.

O'Mahoney, P. D. (1982). Psychiatric denial of mental illness as a normal process. *British Journal of Medical Psychology, 55,* 109–118.

Parker, G. (1982). Re-searching the schizophrenogenic mother. *Journal of Nervous and Mental Disease, 170,* 452–462.

Paulson, R. (1991). Professional training for consumers and family members. *Psychosocial Rehabilitation Journal, 14,* 69–80.

Pearlin, L. I., & Schooler, C. (1978). The structure of coping. *Journal of Health and Science Behavior, 19,* 2–12.

Penn, D. (1991). Cognitive rehabilitation of social defects in schizophrenia: A direction of promise or following a primrose path? *Psychosocial Rehabilitation Journal, 15,* 27–41.

Pepper, B., & Ryglewicz, H. (1986). The stimulus window: Stress and stimulation as aspects of everyday experience. *Tie Lines, 3,* 1–4.

Pilvin, B. (1982). And wisdom to know the difference. In H. Shetler & P.

Straw. (Eds.), *A new day: Voices from across the land* (pp. 21–24). Arlington, VA: National Alliance for the Mentally Ill.

Plath, S. (1977). *Letters home: Correspondence 1950–63* (A. Plath, Ed.). New York: Bantam.

Rabkin, J. (1984). Community attitudes and local facilities. In J. Talbott (Ed.), *The chronic mental patient: Five years later* (pp. 325–335). New York: Grune & Stratton.

Reiser, M. (1988). Are psychiatric educators "losing the mind"? *American Journal of Psychiatry, 145,* 148–153.

Rippere, V., & Williams, R. (1985). *Wounded healers: Mental health workers' experiences of depression.* New York: Wiley.

Robey K., Coen, B., & Gara, M. (1989). Self structure in schizophrenia. *Journal of Abnormal Psychology, 98,* 436–442.

Rutter, M. (1986). Meyerian psychobiology, personality development, and the role of life experiences. *American Journal of Psychiatry, 143,* 1077–1087.

Sabshin, M. (1990). Turning points in twentieth century psychiatry. *American Journal of Psychiatry, 147,* 1267–1274.

Sarason, S. B. (1985). *Caring and compassion in clinical practice.* San Francisco: Jossey-Bass.

Savelson, L. (1986). *I'm not crazy, I just lost my glasses.* Berkeley, CA: DeNova Press.

Schwartz, M., & Wiggins, O. (1985). Science, humanism, and the nature of medical practice: A phenomenological view. *Perspectives in Biology and Medicine, 28,* 331–361.

Sechehaye, M. (1951). *Autobiography of a schizophrenic girl.* New York: New American Library.

Selye, H. (1976). *The stress of life* (rev. ed.). New York: McGraw-Hill.

Selzer, M.A., Sullivan, T. B., Carsky, M., & Terkelsen, K. G. (1989). *Working with the person with schizophrenia: The treatment alliance.* New York: New York University Press.

Sharp, M. L. (1987, Spring). Schizophrenia — how it feels. *Newsletter of the Alliance for the Mentally Ill of Tucson and Southern Arizona,* p. 1.

Sherman, P. S. & Porter, R. (1991). Mental health consumers as case management aides. *Hospital and Community Psychiatry. 42,* 494–498.

Shetler, H., & Straw, P. (Eds.). (1982). *A new day: Voices from across the land.* Arlington, VA: National Alliance for the Mentally Ill.

Shweder, R. A., & Bourne, E. J. (1982). Does the concept of the person vary cross-culturally? In A. J. Marsella & G. M. White (Eds.), *Cultural conceptions of mental health and therapy* (pp. 97–137). Dordrecht, The Netherlands: D. Reidel.

Slater, E. (1989). A parent's view on enforcing medication. In National Alliance for the Mentally Ill, *The experiences of patients and families: First person accounts reprinted from Schizophrenia Bulletin and the New York Times.* Arlington, VA: NAMI.

Smoyak, S. (Ed.). (1975). *The psychiatric nurse as a family therapist.* New York: Wiley.

Snavely, W. (1989). Foreword. In National Alliance for the Mentally Ill, *The experiences of patients and families: First person accounts reprinted from Schizophrenia Bulletin and the New York Times* (p. v). Arlington, VA: NAMI.

Sommer, R., & Osmond, H. (1960). Autobiographies of former mental patients. *Journal of Mental Science, 106,* 648–660.

Sommer, R., & Osmond, H. (1961). Autobiographies of former mental patients. *Journal of Mental Science, 107,* 1030–1032.

Sommers, I. (1987). Tolerance of deviance and the community adjustment of the mentally ill. *Community Mental Health Journal, 23,* 159–182.

Spohn, H., Coyne, L., Larson, J., Mittleman, F., Spray, J. & Hayes, K. (1986). Episodic and residual thought pathology in chronic schizophrenics: Effects of nueroleptics. *Schizophrenic Bulletin, 12,* 394–407.

Spring, B. (1981). Stress and schizophrenia: Some definitional issues. *Schizophrenia Bulletin, 7,* 24–33.

Strachan, A. A. (1986). Family intervention for the rehabilitation of schizophrenia: Toward protection and coping. *Schizophrenia Bulletin, 12,* 678–698.

Strauss, J. S. (1986). Discussion: What does rehabilitation accomplish? *Schizophrenia Bulletin, 12,* 720–723.

Strauss, J. S. (1987). The role of the patient in recovery from psychosis. In J. S. Strauss, W. Boken, & H. Brenner (Eds.), *Psychosocial treatment of schizophrenia* (pp. 160–166). Toronto: Hans Huber.

Strauss, J. S. (1989a). Mediating processes in schizophrenia. *British Journal of Psychiatry, 155,* 22–28.

Strauss, J. S. (1989b). Subjective experiences of schizophrenia: Toward a new dynamic psychiatry. *Schizophrenia Bulletin, 15,* 179–188.

Strauss, J. S., & Carpenter, W. T. (1981). *Schizophrenia.* New York: Plenum Press.

Strauss, J. S., & Estroff, S. E. (1989). Foreword. *Schizophrenia Bulletin, 15,* 177–178.

Strauss, J. S., Harding, C., Hafez, H., & Lieberman, P. (1987). The role of the patient in recovery from psychosis. In J. S. Strauss & W. Boker (Eds.), *Psychosocial treatment of schizophrenia.* Toronto: Hans Huber.

Stuve, P., Erickson, R. C., & Spaulding, W. (1991). Cognitive rehabilitation: The next step in psychiatric rehabilitation. *Psychosocial Rehabilitation Journal, 14,* 5–26.

Styron, W. (1990). *Darkness visible.* New York: Random House.

Sullivan, W. P., & Poertner, J. (1989). Social support and life stress: A mental health consumers perspective. *Community Mental Health Journal, 25,* 21–32.

Susko, M. A. (Ed.). (1991). *Cry of the invisible.* Baltimore: Conservatory Press.

Swan, R. W., & Lavitt, M. R. (1986). *Patterns of adjustment to violence in families of the mentally ill.* New Orleans: Elizabeth Wisner Research center, Tulane University School of Social Work.

Terkelsen, K. G. (1983). Schizophrenia and the family: II. Adverse effects of family therapy. *Family Process, 22,* 191–200.

Torrey, E. F. (1983). *Surviving schizophrenia: A family manual.* New York: Harper & Row.

Torrey, E. F. (1988). *Surviving schizophrenia: A family manual* (rev. ed.). New York: Harper & Row.

Unger, K. V., Anthony, W. A. Sciarappa, K., & Rogers, E. S. (1991). A supported education program for young adults with long-term mental illness. *Hospital and Community Psychiatry, 42,* 838–842.

Vaughn, C. E., Snyder, K. S., Jones, S. Freeman, W., & Falloon, I. R. H. (1984). Family factors in schizophrenic relapse. *Archives of General Psychiatry, 41,* 1169–1177.

Vonnegut, M. (1974). Why I want to bite R. D. Laing. *Harper's Magazine,* pp. 90–92.

Vonnegut, M. (1975). *The Eden express: A personal account of schizophrenia.* New York: Praeger.

Wadeson, H., & Carpenter, W. (1976). Subjective experiences of schizophrenia. *Schizophrenia Bulletin, 2,* 302–316.

Warner, R., Taylor, D., Powers, M. & Hyman, J. (1989). Acceptance of the mental illness label by psychotic patients: Effects on functioning. *American Journal of Orthopsychiatry, 59,* 398–409.

Watts, F. N., Powell, G. E., & Austin, S. V. (1975). The modification of abnormal beliefs. *British Journal of Medical Psychology, 46,* 359–363.

Waxler, N. E. (1984). Culture and mental illness: A social labeling perspective. In J. E. Mezzich & C. E. Berganza (Eds.), *Culture and psychopathology* (pp. 556–80). New York: Columbia University Press.

Weiner, S. (1982). Exhaustion and fairness. In H. Shetler & P. Straw (Eds.), *A new day: Voices from across the land* (pp. 9–10). Arlington, VA: National Alliance for the Mentally Ill.

Weiner, S. (1985). We are different: Some thoughts on looking at society and culture. *Hang Tough: Newsletter of the Marin Network of Mental Health Clients, 1*(2), 3.

Weiner, S. (1987). Bravado and the mental health clients' self-help movement. *Hang Tough: Newsletter of the Marin Network of Mental Health Clients, 2*(2), 6.

Weiss, K. M. (1989). Advantages of abandoning symptom-based diagnostic systems of research in schizophrenia. *American Journal of Orthopsychiatry, 59,* 324–330.

Westermeyer, J. (1989). Psychiatric epidemiology across cultures: Current issues and trends. *Transcultural Psychiatric Research Review, 26,* 5–25.

White, R. (1974). Strategies of adaptation: An attempt at systematic description. In G. V. Coelho, D. A. Hamburg, & J. E. Adams (Eds.), *Coping and adaptation* (pp. 47–68). New York: Basic Books.

Zahniser, J., Coursey, R., & Hershberger, B. (1991). Individual psychotherapy with schizophrenic outpatients in the public mental health system. *Hospital and Community Psychiatry, 42,* 906–912.

Zelt, D. (1989). First person account: The Messiah quest. In National Alliance for the Mentally Ill, *The experiences of patients and families: First person accounts reprinted from Schizophrenia Bulletin and the New York Times* (pp. 45–49). Arlington, VA: NAMI.

Index

Acceptance
  by community, 100, 104–113,
    125, 127, 128, 144, 183
  of illness, 25, 134–136, 142, 148,
    154, 162, 165, 184, 185
Accomplishment, sense of, 148–150,
  186
Acting-out behavior, 14, 52
Adaptation
  as process, 132–134
  theory, 13, 15, 16, 25, 40, 177
Adult children of schizophrenics, 83,
  84, 89, 181
Affect, inappropriate, 60–62, 66
Alliance for the Mentally Ill, 111,
  113
American Mental Health Fund, 110
Anger
  adaptive aspects of, 164
  as coping response, 21, 22, 25
  displaced, 84, 106
  provoked, 107
  uncontrollable, 115
Antipsychiatry groups, 107
Antisocial behavior, 82
Anxiety, 30, 56, 57, 66, 153
  management, 57, 62, 66
Apathy, 162; see also Passivity
Arts, 149, 150, 166, 167, 186
Associative connections, 45, 46, 51,
  179
Attention, disorders of, 35–37, 51,
  53, 82, 180
Attribution theory, 13, 16–18, 25
Autonomy, 125, 128, 153, 155, 165
  ambivalence about, 84, 89, 90
  restrictions on, in hospitalization,
    22, 92

B

Behavior
  antisocial, 82
  as coping strategy, 106
  deviant, 146
  and social meaning, 12
Belief modification, 53
Boundaries; see Ego boundaries
Bravado, 136

C

California Well-Being Project, 85, 93,
  95, 96, 98, 101, 103, 166
Chronicity, 10, 25, 108
Cognitive disturbances; see Thought
  disorders
Cognitive therapy, 53
Coherence, 30
Communications, 53, 54, 124
Community acceptance, 100,
  104–113, 125, 127, 128,
  144, 183
Community Care (Denver), 120–122
Concentration; see Attention,
  disorders of
Consumer advocacy groups, 4,
  20–26, 111, 113
  antipsychiatry stance of, 21, 98
  as coping strategy, 22–24, 107
  interaction of with professionals,
    23
  and labeling, 107–109
  leaders of, overwork in, 164, 165
  service models, 22, 23
  and treatment limitations, 165
  writers in, 97, 166

Control, 38, 40, 41, 127
  of attention, 36, 37
  of illness, 122, 142, 155, 165
  illusion of, 84
  locus of, 40
  loss of, 37, 46
Coping strategies, 11, 20–26, 39,
    52, 90, 127, 188
  active, 20, 25
  and appraisal of experience, 16, 21
  of clinicians, 80
  denial as 20, 132
  intropunitive, 21
  major types of, 20
  maladaptive, 106, 107, 112, 132,
    133
  palliative, 132
  versus primary illness mechanisms,
    133
  and societal attitudes, 18
  for stigmatization, 105–109
  theory of, 13, 15, 16
  for thought disorders, 49–51
  training, 39, 121, 123
  withdrawal as, 163, 168
Creative expression, 166, 167
Cultural world view, 13, 17–19, 24,
    25, 80, 85

D

Decompensation, 14, 81, 117, 186
  avoiding, 154, 155
  warning signs of 158–161, 168,
    186
Deinstitutionalization, 163
Delusions, 19, 35, 42, 53, 68, 180
  of control by outside forces, 29,
    37, 46
  as coping efforts, 133
  paranoid, 32, 104, 169, 170
  public perception of, 101
Denial, 5, 21, 108, 136, 142
  as defense mechanism, 20, 106,
    107, 132, 133
  by family, 115
  of illness, 25, 98, 99, 182, 183
Dependency, 84–87, 89, 155
  exaggerated, 166
  and hospitalization, 121
Depression, 46, 56–59, 66, 153
  in mental health professionals, 152

postpsychotic, 143
  public perception of, 101
  symptoms of, 57
Despair, versus hope, 122, 136, 137
Developmental interruption, 84
Deviance hypothesis, 13
Disempowerment, 21
Disengagement, 20, 22

E

Education, 164
  for families, 7, 8, 52, 79, 81, 111
  for patients, 156, 165, 168
  public, 110, 164
  supported, 167, 168
Ego boundaries, 18, 24, 29, 30, 62,
    147, 178
Ego-defense mechanisms, 106, 133,
    145
Emotion-focused coping, 20–22
Emotions; *see* Affect, inappropriate;
    Feelings
Empathy, 3, 4, 6, 10, 83, 183, 187
  lack of, 62
  obstacles to, 7
Employment
  finding, 151
  skills, 122
  stigmatization in 102–105, 110,
    151, 183
  transitional, 110
Empowerment, 22, 125, 126, 188
Engagement, versus meaningless, 153
Engulfment, 5, 40, 178
Entitlement benefits, 104, 112
Environment, 10, 40
  interpersonal, 13, 14, 25, 40; *see
    also* Interpersonal relationships
  order/structure in, 49–51, 54,179
  overstimulating, 162, 163, 186
  supportive, 52, 53
Ethnographic study, 9, 93, 94
Exhibitionism, 106
Expressed emotion (EE), 80–82

F

Families, 79–90, 115, 181, 182,
    187, 188
  as cause of schizophrenia, 13, 39,
    79, 80

education for 7, 8, 52, 79, 81, 111, 119, 123–125
patients' perceptions of, 85–90
stresses in, 81, 82
as support systems, 111, 113, 119, 123, 182
Fear, 56, 83, 171
Feelings, 173; *see also* Affect, inappropriate
intense, 147
interpreting, 63, 66
of loss, in siblings, 83
Fellowship House, 110
Friendship, 64, 170, 185

G

Games, 149
Grandiosity, 34, 101, 106, 155
Guilt
inappropriate, 59, 60
in parents, 84–87, 90
in siblings, 83

H

Hallucinations, 19, 35, 46, 48, 53, 180
auditory, 15, 117, 160–162, 168, 171
as coping efforts, 133
public perception of, 101
Healing, 152, 184, 186
Helplessness; *see* Powerlessness
Hobbies, 149, 186
Homeless mentally ill, 100
Homeostatic control, 10
Hope, 122, 136, 137, 141, 154, 185
Hospitalization, 5, 22, 72–75, 84, 91, 118
as countertherapeutic, 93, 119–121
and identity, 112
patient–staff relationships in, 92, 96
and powerlessness, 106
survey on, 98
William Styron on, 96
Housing
stigmatization in, 102, 111, 183
supported, 163
Humor, 165

I

Identity, 6, 9, 25, 30, 144, 183
acceptable obstacles to achieving, 144–148
confusion about, 147
disruption of, 5, 19, 29, 33, 34
as patient, 24, 112, 127, 143, 185
recovery as threat to, 147
and social rejection, 145, 185
statements, 10
and work, 150
in young people, 153, 185
Independence; *see* Autonomy
Independence Center (St. Louis), 141, 170, 172
Interdependence, 87, 90
Interpersonal relationships, 63–66, 114, 119–128, 185
in the community, 125–128
in families, 123–125
with mental health professionals, 119–122, 141, 185
sensitivity in, 119, 180
Intimacy, 63, 153
Isolation; *see* Withdrawal

J

Judgment, 49

L

Labeling, 9, 24, 108, 109, 134, 142, 145
internalized, 25
theory, 5, 17
Laing, R. D., 97
Legal accountability, 17
Life events
research, 13, 25, 160
as stressors, 15, 160
Listening, 6, 41
Loneliness, 62–65, 147

M

"Madness–badness" dichotomy, 17, 25
Mania, 42, 43, 46, 60
Manipulation, 106

Meaning, 143, 183, 184, 186
ways of finding, 147–150
Medication, 20, 40, 65, 91, 101,
121, 178
attitudes toward, 94–96
and depression, 57
education about, 156
extrapyramidal effects of, 164
and hallucinations, 15
monitoring, 158, 168
and thought disorders, 42
Memory, 50, 51, 53, 180
Mental health consumer movement;
see Consumer advocacy groups
Mental health system, 151, 187; see
also Hospitalization;
Treatment
and consumer groups, 113; see
also Consumer advocacy
groups
and entitlement benefits, 104
paternalism in, 92
patients' perceptions of, 21–24,
91–99, 128, 141
as stressor, 20, 22
training for, 7, 152
Mood disorders, 55, 57
Mothers, schizophrenogenic, 80; see
also Families

N

National Alliance for the Mentally
Ill, 8, 82, 110, 166
Siblings and Adult Children
Network, 83
National Art Exhibitions by the
Mentally Ill, Inc., 166, 167
National Association of Psychiatric
Survivors, 91, 107
National Consumers Conference, 67,
68
National Mental Health Consumers'
Association, 98, 107, 108
Neuropsychology, 53
Neurotransmitter dysfunction, 14, 25
Noncompliance, 6, 65, 82, 156, 158

O

Objectivity, 7, 177
Observation, clinical, 5, 41

Obsession, 116
Overinclusiveness, 43

P

Paranoid ideation, 16, 32, 82, 104,
165, 169–171
and brain dysfunction, 14
self-monitoring for, 168
Passivity, 5, 37, 178
Patient reports, 8, 177, 178
Patterns, of discontinuity, 133, 184
Pejorative language, 107–109, 112,
120
Perceptions; see also Self-perception
conflicting, 32
distorted, 30, 48, 117
of mentally ill; see Stigmatization
of recovery process, 184
Personal documents, 9
Phenomenology, 4, 6
Picture drawing, 9
Plath, Sylvia, 87
Poetry, 150
Powerlessness, 22, 40, 106, 126,
179
in parents, 85
Prejudice, 109, 111, 112; see also
Stigmatization
Problem-focused coping, 20, 25
Program for Assertive Community
Treatment (PACT), 93, 94,
110
Projection, 106, 133
Prolixin, 94, 95, 170
Psychodynamic therapy, 11, 87, 88,
90, 121, 155, 182
Psychosis, 6, 11, 14, 19, 185; see
also Schizophrenia
cyclical nature of, 104, 160, 186
disturbed perceptions in, 30
heightened awareness in, 34
investment in, 143
as loss of boundaries, 19
stress in, 30, 160, 178
subliminal processes in, 54
thought disorders in, 42, 43

R

Readaptation, 132, 133, 184
Reality testing, 124

Reasoning, 48
Recovery, 128, 131, 137, 140–142,
    172, 173, 179
  as adaptation, 133
  discontinuity in, 133, 184
  factors in, 134–141, 184
  and stigmatization, 104
  study of, 171
  symbols of, 131
Recovery, Inc., 165
Rehabilitation, 6, 20, 39, 66, 140,
    155
  and community acceptance, 110,
    111, 113
  and institutionalization, 93
  psychosocial, 6, 121, 133, 141,
    182, 183
  staff attitudes in, 140
Relapse; *see* Decompensation
Residential treatment, 120–122
Resocialization, 20
Responsibility, versus victimization,
    135, 136, 143
Rogers, Joe, 98
Role diffusion, 144

S

Scale for the Assessment of Negative
    Symptoms, 62
Schizophrenia, 3, 11, 12, 19, 30,
    180
  as biopsychosocial phenomenon,
    13, 25
  chronic, 15, 17, 19, 24
  as identity, 30, 37, 147
  and interpersonal environment, 13,
    14, 25, 40
  media attention to, 109, 110, 113
  as stressor, 11, 13, 15
  thought processes in, example of,
    67–76
Security, need for, 128
Self
  boundaries; *see* Ego boundaries
  defenses focusing on, 21
  disturbed perception of, 29, 30,
    33–35, 40, 147, 178
  loss of, 19, 30, 37, 178, 185
  and social identity, 33
Self-behavior management strategies,
    156–168

Self-concept, 5, 12
Self-diagnosis, 156
Self-esteem
  and grandiosity, 106
  impaired, 62, 92, 100
  increased, 121, 127, 141, 155,
    167
Self-Help Center (St. Louis County),
    173, 174
Self-help groups, 22, 23, 98, 126,
    127, 138, 165
Self-monitoring, 154, 155, 157,
    165, 168
Self-perception
  and community acceptance, 100,
    104–109, 112
  and other mentally ill patients,
    145, 146
Self theory, 13, 18
Selye, Hans, 13, 14
Semantic strategies, 24
Shaman, 152
Shame, 21, 83
Siblings, 82–84, 89, 115, 119,
    181
Skill building, 20, 39, 52, 121, 122,
    133, 155
Social isolation, 163; *see also*
    Withdrawal
Social rejection, 146, 147, 184
Social retardation, 84, 90, 171, 173,
    185
Social role, 13, 19, 144
Social support systems, 138–140; *see*
    also Self-help groups
Specialized Mental Health Training
    Program (Cincinnati, Ohio),
    152
Stigmatization, 24, 83, 100–113,
    126, 128, 145, 146, 183, 184;
    see also Social rejection
  coping with, 105–109, 123
  in employment, 102–105, 110,
    112
  in housing, 102, 111, 112
  internalization of 104, 105, 112,
    146
  and medicalization, 110
Stimulation, 51–54, 81, 162, 163,
    186; *see also* Expressed
    emotion
Stimulus barrier, 51

Stress, 13–16, 153
and coping strategies, 20–25, 127,
163
and psychosis, 30, 104, 160, 178
and stimulation, 52
and thought disorders, 49, 51
Styron, William, 96, 97
Subjective experience, 5, 160, 177,
178
role of in research, 8–10, 177
Substance abuse, 52, 154, 170
Support groups; *see* Self-help groups;
Social support systems

T

Therapists, free choice of, 96
Thought disorders, 42–54, 133, 179,
180; *see also* Delusions
blocking, 47, 51
coping strategies for, 49–51, 179
loss of meaning in, 47, 48
racing thoughts, 83, 43–46, 51,
179
slowed thought, 46, 47, 179
Thought–behavior connection, 8
Treatment, 91, 118, 182; *see also*
Hospitalization; Medication;
Rehabilitation
cooperation in, 39

individualized, 128
involuntary, 165
negative, 119, 120
Trust, 119, 121, 141, 172, 185

U

Understanding; *see* Empathy
Usefulness, 150–152, 186

V

Values, traditional, 140
Violence, 82
Voices; *see* Hallucinations, auditory
Vulnerability–stress–coping–
competence model, 52

W

Ways of Coping Scale, 20
Withdrawal, 52, 106, 115, 116, 125
and adaptation, 133, 163, 168

Y

Yalom, I. D., 153